T0196124

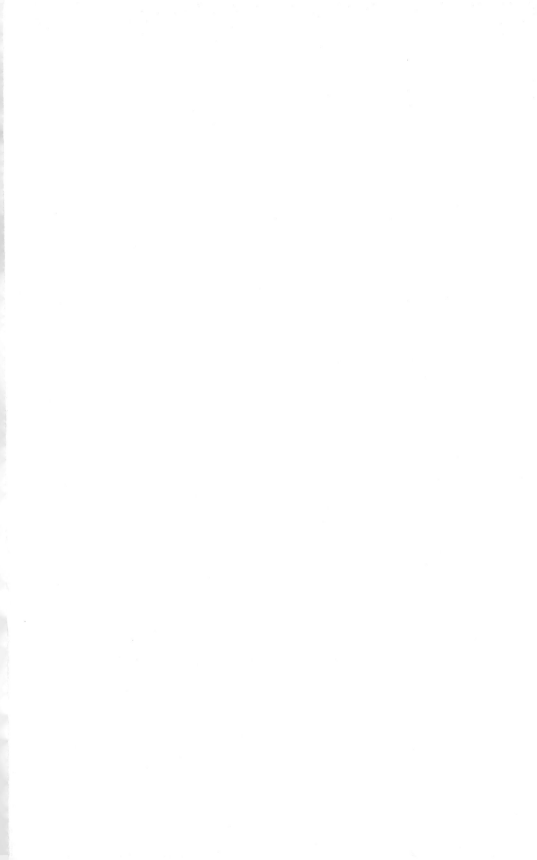

# BREAKING OUT OF THE HEALTH CARE ABYSS

## TRANSFORMATIONAL TIPS FOR AGENTS OF CHANGE

ROYER-MADDOX-HERRON

authorHOUSE®

*AuthorHouse*™
*1663 Liberty Drive*
*Bloomington, IN 47403*
*www.authorhouse.com*
*Phone: 1 (800) 839-8640*

*Published by AuthorHouse  08/24/2017*

*ISBN: 978-1-5246-7209-6 (sc)*
*ISBN: 978-1-5246-7210-2 (hc)*
*ISBN: 978-1-5246-7208-9 (e)*

*Library of Congress Control Number: 2017902596*

*Print information available on the last page.*

*This book is printed on acid-free paper.*

# Contents

# Foreword

## By Pat Keel, FHFMA

I am honored to write this forward. This is an exceptional book that comes timely on the heels of many disruptions and changes in the healthcare environment. The landscape of healthcare is evolving at such a rapid pace that it is difficult to plan for the future. The level and complexity of change in the environment requires that we, as leaders, also evolve. I am delighted to have this insightful text on how to leverage change, especially during times of turbulence. This book is especially perceptive because it is authored by a trio of men for whom I have the highest level of respect and confidence, and men that I know have succeeded in this type of environment. I have had the pleasure of working with Tom Royer M.D., Peter Maddox, and Jay Herron for seven years during periods of dramatic change in our organization. Jay Herron has been a mentor for me for over 15 years, and his influence has been contributory to many of my professional changes. I have seen first-hand how these healthcare leaders have used change—even disruptive change—to transform organizations to stronger, more flexible and innovative organizations.

# Prologue

# Caution: Turbulence Ahead

We, the authors, collectively have more than 100 years of hospital leadership experience in some of the most recognized healthcare organizations in the United States. Additionally, we worked as a team for 13 years responding to leadership/governance/management challenges in the U.S. and abroad. During our careers, we have continually encountered situations where people seemingly know what to do and yet for some unexplained reason, implementation is lacking. This causes us to be concerned. This book is a warning to boards and leaders of hospital organizations, and other related industries, of turbulent conditions ahead. It is also a book that challenges the established paradigms of many governance and leaders in hospitals and related organizations. In times of turbulence existing management concepts, patterns of behavior and expectations for future results will need to be reimagined and reengineered (Imagineering comes to mind as a critical success factor) for success. Joel A. Barker, futurist, author and strategist has often referred to the transition from established paradigms to new models as a "paradigm shift". His research has shown that truly dramatic paradigm shifts most often are not led by those in established organizations because they have too much at stake to upset the status quo. (1)

Assumptions that have impacted hospital decision making for the past 40 years are dramatically changing. Bigger is better, volumes will increase, technology gets more expensive, doctors will always be autonomous, surgery will always be done in a hospital, people prefer to have a personal relationship with a doctor, etc. The future includes patients being forced to become healthcare customers that shop for the services they need.

Venture capitalists will fund real innovators creating companies disruptive to the healthcare status quo. These can be seen particularly in technology applications that promise to improve lives or at the very least, provide pathways through the morass of the healthcare system. Home health, which is not adequately reimbursed by private or government payers, still promises to grow and to provide a clear alternative to traditional health care delivery sites. Government policy makers will rely on transparency and fund pilot programs to improve quality and cost as value replaces volume as a primary business metric. Such programs will rely heavily on reimbursement/payment incentives because that is the government paradigm for driving change. And, because of this, there is one thing we are absolutely positive about: reimbursement for health care providers will decline.

In this state of transition, health care is big news. The media is reporting stories to illustrate issues within the current healthcare system. Authors are exploring the topic, as evidenced in recent book titles like: "The Patient Will See You Now, The Future of Medicine is in Your Hands;" "The Creative Destruction of Medicine, How the Digital Revolution Will Create Better Health Care;" "Catastrophic Care: How American Health Care Killed My Father-And How We Can Fix It;" "America's Bitter Pill: Money, Politics, Backroom Deals, and the Fight to Fix our Broken Healthcare System;" "The Patient's Playbook: How to Save Your Life and the Lives of Those You Love;" "The Digital Doctor;" and "Reinventing American Health Care: How the Affordable Care Act Will Improve our Terribly Complex, Blatantly Unjust, Outrageously Expensive, Grossly Inefficient, Error Prone System."

Perhaps the most indicting analysis is a series of patient safety studies over the last two decades. In an often cited and landmark study reported in 1999 by the Institute of Medicine, deaths due to medical errors were said to be up to 99,000 per year. Even though the study, To Err Is Human, stated that this figure could be on the low end, the American medical community accepted this number as real and, more importantly, said that something must be done. Great efforts were put in place to measure, improve and account for medical harm. (2)

Sadly, the New England Journal of Medicine reported in a follow up study on deaths and adverse events between 2002 and 2007 that patient safety did not improve.(3) In 2010, the Office of the Inspector General for Health and Human Services published an estimate that as many as 180,000 people were dying because of adverse events in hospitals.(4) In 2013, a NASA based toxicologist, John James PhD, published a study using data from 2008-2011 (subsequent assessments of his methods were confirmed by four different statisticians) in which he estimated as many as 440,000 patients were dying from preventable adverse events.(5) In 2016, Johns Hopkins University School of Medicine researchers published yet another study that identified as many 250,000 deaths each year that can be attributed to medical mistakes. (6) These studies have identified a problem of immense concern.

It is outrageous that this is occurring. It is known that we have a problem in this country. The US healthcare *non-system* is simply not as effective as it should be, especially when compared with other first-world countries. The US healthcare system is expensive and is estimated to cost almost 50 percent more than the next nearest country when care is measured on a per capita basis. (7) And, sadly, we have poorer health outcomes to go along with this spending. Knowing is clearly not enough. Action is sorely lacking.

It is difficult to understand the momentum of this downward spiral, given the vast amount of knowledge and resources available in books, journals, magazines, articles, undergraduate and graduate hospital administration programs, leadership seminars, trade organizations and development programs. While healthcare is recognized as a complex industry, the research and guidance that is available to leaders to improve its performance has gone for naught. Is the healthcare industry approaching a tipping point?

(8) In recent history, we've witnessed the bankruptcy of General Motors, a country-wide real estate crisis, a global financial crisis and a greater than 70 percent decline in the price of a barrel of crude oil. Apparently, it's difficult to predict when tipping points will occur. Here are some nominees:

- American healthcare in 2016 was a $3 trillion financial juggernaut. (9) The financing of the industry is largely opaque to the general public. But transparency is rapidly developing. Healthcare consumes 18% of GDP (up from 8% in the '50s). Will the tipping point be at 20%, 25%?
- The Internet makes mass communication of issues easier. Healthcare information is becoming more accessible. Will information, public education and knowledge be the tipping point?
- Until recently, the largest segments of the population, the elderly and employed people, have been insulated from the financial risks of illness through Medicare and employer provided health insurance. For these groups, access to healthcare and the cost of healthcare have been non-issues. These traditional types of benefits are changing and as they do more, questions will be asked about how the delivery system works. An example of change is Medicare Advantage programs. These are growing in number. They provide additional services and lower out-of-pocket costs than traditional Medicare (as long as the beneficiary is willing to accept restrictions on providers and some other services and limits to their coverage areas). The Accountable Care Act of 2010 has provided Medicaid up to 200% of the Federal Poverty Level (in states that expanded Medicaid), eliminating out of pocket costs for the poor and dual-eligible Medicare patient. While these changes mentioned above are put forth in U.S. government regulations, these can be changed by executive and/or Congressional action. We believe there are benefit changes that will be more permanent due to obvious cost savings. These are found in the commercial sector. Employers are changing plans in various ways to include higher deductibles, limitations on coverage and increased premiums. Some employers have gone so far as to provide a fixed amount "health care voucher" for employees to use to purchase their own self/family coverage

and, thereby, getting the employer out of the de facto provision of coverage and most clearly out of the headaches of managing a complex benefit. (10)

Experience can be a harsh, but oftentimes, very good teacher. Unfortunately, for healthcare leaders, there haven't been very many industry-wide crises to provide learning opportunities. Each of us at Royer Maddox Herron Advisors was involved in healthcare organizations during the major disruptive policy change of 1984, The Prospective Payment System. This plan converted the Medicare program from a "cost reimbursed" system (the more you spend, the more you get "reimbursed") to a prospectively determined payment system (fixed payments for hospital stays via predetermined Diagnosis Related Groups, or DRGs). Commercial insurers followed the federal government lead thus ensuring that these changes were essentially nationwide. This set in motion significant changes in how medicine would be paid and therefore altered how medicine was practiced, and, thereby, how hospitals would need to operate differently in the future. One major result of the DRG system of payment was that lengths of stays dropped precipitously, in some cases by as much as half. This change created massive excess capacity forcing hospital leaders to figure out how to convert facilities to other uses or close the space and lay off healthcare workers. A significant number of hospitals completely closed because of the inability to adapt to the new environment. Many organizations began to lose money caring for Medicare patients. This, along with dramatic improvements in anesthesiology and other technical improvements as well as certain payment incentives, helped to stimulate the migration from inpatient services to outpatient services.

Lessons learned from what happened to our organizations remain top of mind for us.

Today's healthcare environment is undergoing subtle changes comparable to those of the Prospective Payment era. Will there be a healthcare crisis? We believe there already is a healthcare crisis. Or multiple crises. There is too much money in the healthcare system. This is due to high prices for many services and even higher prices for drugs. The crisis is too much money that, in an ironic twist, "insulates" professionals from scrutiny and questioning. The crisis is in class roles occupied by physicians and leaders. The crisis is in technology developed, acquired and, therefore, used, often-times, ill advisedly and too frequently. The crisis is in consumers who are sheltered from the real cost of the care that they receive. The crisis is in a system of quality reviews that are all too often subjectively based, done by peers of the professional being reviewed and lack significant consequences for misbehavior or mistakes.

In the meantime, employers are changing healthcare benefit plans requiring employees to make their own choices for their healthcare decisions. The unintended consequence is to make healthcare users ask better questions and become better healthcare consumers. But, in truth, the real driver of this is to lower employer costs. The Centers for Medicare & Medicaid Services are piloting programs to improve care and quality for patients and lower the cost of services. Numerous studies have disclosed massive amounts of waste in the current delivery system. (11) What will be the impact of taking these costs out of the system? Removing waste, rework and redundancy actually reduces provider incomes, which exposes the perverse incentives of fee-for-service payments. Private employers and the federal government represent the two largest payment sources for healthcare. As more documentation becomes available outlining opportunities for savings through eliminating unnecessary rework, government and private funding sources will lower total payments to providers. In the last several decades the healthcare industry has benefitted from an endless increase in funding since the beginning of the Medicare program in 1965. How extensive the healthcare environment will be impacted by the cumulative impact of changes in health insurance, increased transparency, a consumer orientation and value based outcomes is unknown. We believe providers that have the knowledge, but wait to react to the impact, will most likely be in jeopardy. Not to mention the ones that are clueless.

The role of every healthcare leader is to navigate their organization through turbulent times. Situational awareness is the first obligation of effective leaders. The courage and will to make necessary change, no matter how difficult or challenging, is the second. Today's environment is calling for courageous leaders. Times of chaos enable greater opportunities for knowledge development. Improving patient care, improving quality and lowering costs are fundamental to organizations' survival. Indeed, it may be fundamental to the survival of the entire American medical experience. It will take courage, confidence and capability to implement transformational behaviors as organizational cultures are inherently resistant to change. It will take innovative, bold leaders to guide people through transformational changes to transcend the challenges.

Let's cut to the chase:

Healthcare is a big mess, impossible to fully understand, much less control.

The literature is awash with guidance, much of it contradictory; full of "conventional wisdom" and so you can find support for any answer you like.

This book cuts through the clutter and presents a clear path for navigating the whitewater ahead.

# Chapter I

# The Journey of Transformation

**"Change is the law of life. And those who look only to the past or present are certain to miss the future." -- John F. Kennedy**

**The Journey of Transformation**

We are all on a journey. It never ends. Every day along this path there are transitions. Every step we take is a movement placing us someplace new.

Most transitions are incremental. Transitions can be so small that we may not even notice them. On the other hand, transformation can be monumental. It is far beyond a transition, and therefore, far more impactful. It is a major change. It is to become something else. Like the caterpillar to the butterfly.

Transformation can occur suddenly, or slowly over an extended period. Major transformations are all around us. They are a part of our lives, culture, values, country, organizations, employment and environments. If a major change happens relatively quickly it can be indelibly imprinted upon our minds. Sudden change is immediately realized as impactful. Incremental change, which is not so sudden and indeed may take years to be realized, can be equally impactful but may not be noticed. If we pause to look back and reflect, we are aware of the significance of the change. So, reflection, and even introspection, can be a valued aspect of understanding transformation.

## An Indelible Transformative Moment in History

An example of this latter type of transformation occurred at the time of the assassination of President Kennedy. This egregious act was transformational in its own way. It was tragic, shocking and riveting. It was the end of the American Camelot. It was the beginning of a string of assassinations and murderous attempts at some of our most respected idols. It changed much about how we interact with our leaders. But, there was another transformation that occurred at President Kennedy's death. Media consumption.

Prior to the day our nation watched the black and white replays of Jackie enveloping a collapsed JFK in Dallas, or John-John's salute at his father's funeral, we tuned in to black and white newsprint.

Everyone followed current events from a newspaper. One of the authors of this book, Peter, had a grandfather who was a journalist, and taught journalism for 40 years. He was proud of the printed word. News had been shared this way for centuries, since the advent of the printing press. As Americans were glued to TV sets to understand the unthinkable, it was the beginning of the decline for newspapers. While his grandfather was a friend of television newscasters, he saw the new medium as simply an additional type of communication in the journalistic armamentarium. He missed the transformative impact of countrywide television broadcasts. He never saw the shift from regionally based communication to one more national in scope.

What happened that day in Dallas affected all Americans. And the world. It helped reshape how we not only received information, but also how we processed it and understood it. From a linguistics standpoint, network broadcasting helped diminish our regional differences in speech and language and interpretation. In short, television news helped to usher in changes to the national culture itself. For those born since the assassination of President Kennedy these changes are not a change; but they are-in fact- a transformative moment, a historical moment, now made into a new reality.

Change is a part of life. As important and as subtle as the shift to the TV screen may have been, transformational events have surrounded us; and they continue subtly as well as dramatically. TV moved from the airwaves to cable and now to the internet. The internet itself has transformed communication and connection to each other in countless ways, but particularly through what is called 'social media'. Changes are ever present…and coming at ever increasing numbers and accelerating rates and frequency. From McDonald's first fast food diner to the advent of the "pill," we respond to our primal needs in ways that may have been considered alien to our ancestors. But we respond.

## From the Flush Toilet to the Polio Vaccine

Medical care is no exception, and since the dawn of the 20th Century its evolution has been exponential. The changes in medical care are almost too numerous to mention. Most have been due to technical improvements in anesthesia, pharmaceuticals, surgical techniques and tools, vaccines and increased genetic understanding.

But, interestingly enough, more lives have been saved by two, now totally ignored albeit technical developments: the flush toilet and potable water. These advances are perhaps the greatest generators of health in this country…if not the world. Today, our society takes clean drinking water and sewer systems for granted. The same with extraordinary medical treatments. We too are now taking these for granted. As a result, we believe we are invincible and modern medicine can save us from every calamity. A medical miracle system for some, but a costly quagmire for others. Unfortunately, most of us still have an acute disease mindset in a chronic disease world. We can "cure" acute disease but we cannot "cure" chronic disease; we can diagnose it earlier, slow it down and palliate the symptoms, but not cure.

Indirectly, this cultural shift in attitude may have contributed to the significant funds that have flowed into medical technology and medical research. The medical community shares some culpability for this cultural shift as characterized by the reliance on drugs versus lifestyle modifications. As Pogo said, "We have met the enemy and he is us."

Over the past several decades, there have been many transformations in the healthcare arena. Post WW II, driven by the Baby Boom, the Hill-Burton Act started a building boom in hospitals. Employer-based health insurance coverage followed and medical schools grew in number and size to support the need for qualified medical staff. The establishment of Medicare and Medicaid as major sources of payment for medical services was a significant milestone in the provision of medical services for the elderly and the poor. These two payment systems dramatically influenced how payment formulas developed for similar services, but different populations, by commercial insurance carriers. Structural changes to delivery systems (the alphabet soup of IPAs, HMOs, MSOs, PHOs, IDSs, etc.) in the 1970s and 1980s foreshadowed the focus in the next millennium on access, quality, lower costs and higher efficiencies.

**Agents of Change**

We at Royer-Maddox-Herron Advisors have seen a lot. We were successful because we learned to use every change to create advantage for our institutions. But, learning to manage the growing rulebook of health care in the U.S. is not sufficient. Later in our careers we paused long enough to look beyond our own institutions and take stock of the direction the world around us was heading. We discovered that it was spiraling in a different manner and direction than we had planned and imagined. We realized that our primary duty was not to extract advantage from every minor change in management, payment or technology, but to intentionally transform our organizations for long-term sustainability in a new environment. This had to be done to sustain and even bring increased value to the communities in which we lived and served. But, as we discovered, timing is everything: an organization can be derailed by moving too soon (the "pioneers" are the ones with the arrows in their backs) as moving too late.

Leading is more than just responding to events, opportunities and challenges. It is also looking beyond the exigencies of the moment. Leaders must recognize the drivers and events, from the very subtle to a maelstrom that will sculpt the future landscape. Leaders must foresee what implication the future may bring and make the hard choices necessary to ensure the organizational mission and purpose are sustained. Great leaders make these choices well before the need for them is obvious. Success comes to those who are prepared. Anticipatory intelligence and change behaviors are perhaps the most distinguishing marks of leaders who will be successful in any future environment. Couple these two characteristics with the willingness to abandon practices that brought past success and an organization will find itself blessed with a leader capable of leading it successfully into a new and dynamic future environment.

How does one prepare for a future that, almost by definition, is unknowable? How could a newspaper executive in the 1960s have been able to foreshadow events to prepare for the introduction of the television and the internet? Likewise, how can health care executives become agents of change to foresee dramatically evolving health care services? This book is designed to answer these questions.

**The Current Reality**

The American way of delivering health care and medical care is a complex array of services, agencies, approaches, and personal experiences. Medical care is primarily curative (for acute disease, accidents, etc.) and geared for a sudden onset of illness. The US hospital industry is great at "rescue medicine"! Now, increasingly, medical care encompasses continuing and chronic effects of illness. The majority of services provided in today's hospital are for chronic conditions. Yet, chronic services can be more efficiently addressed in less costly environments than in a hospital. The most effective approach to good health is not medical care at all: it's health promotion and illness prevention. And, it should therefore be obvious, that this is not the purview of the traditional hospital or health care provider. Hospital based organizational leaders need to pay attention... the leadership and authority position now occupied by doctors and hospital executives will likely shift, albeit slowly, to those knowledgeable in illness prevention, health promotion and public health.

Acute care and chronic care, as important as they are for the people in need of them, have little to do with overall health. Let's face it; the most important aspect of any national model to improve health and well-being is the public health system. Any country is healthier with increased standards for proper food handling, sanitation, safety regulations, housing, immunization requirements, nutrition and health education. Today, Social Determinants of Health, a term that came from the book: Social Determinants of Health: The Solid Facts, is used to describe the many different social variables that influence health, including social, political, educational attainment, violence and employment status and economic standard of living. (12) Even with the knowledge that as much as 80% of health status is dependent upon the social determinants of health (13), most of the money and the attention still go to episodic and acute medical care, which is a small part of determining the health status of a community and an even smaller part of the overall health status of the United States. Institutions, organizations and health systems have been well positioned and successful over the past 100 years because of the power of modern medicine and the money that has flowed into its growth and influence. The winds of major transformational events are stirring and growing in strength. Fighting fires once they break out is important, but it is best to prevent them in the first place. A paradigm shift is needed and, we believe, is on the way.

Most organizations think of themselves as capable of handling whatever may come to them. Indeed, the past has shown this to be the case. Unfortunately in health care, institutional change comes slowly. Jay spoke recently at a national conference attended by thousands of the nation's senior healthcare industry leaders. It was his sad observation that little progress in creative response to challenge has occurred and he concluded that there is a vast void in anticipatory thinking among some leaders.

At this meeting, he noted an abundance of 'happy talk', in his words. Economic survival was the underlying theme. There was no mention of the impact of consumerism (something we identified in 2008 as a major transformational change which would grow and become a driving force). There was no mention of transparency and institutional responsibility to the communities in which the institutions were located. There was not even substantive dialogue about plans to improve real or perceived value (higher quality at lower overall cost). The two primary attention grabbers were formulas to maximize payment and a newly designed patient gown.

## Nibbling at the Margin

To be fair, many leadership teams are exploring models that will position their health care organizations for a different future. Most of what is now going on, however, is repositioning for change that has already happened. Most are simply trying to adapt to the new rules of the game. The Patient Protection and Affordable Care Act (ACA) has redefined payment formulas, quality standards and access requirements for all providers. Additionally, the ACA now enables patients and consumers to have more influence. Interestingly, as valuable as the ACA has been in terms of reducing overall costs, improving access for millions of previously uninsured people and establishing higher quality standards, there exists a public perception that the law has caused too much turmoil, something the author Clayton Christensen would call disruptive innovation. Insurance companies positioned themselves to be successful in this new environment. And, there is now occurring a recognition that consumers have real opinions, real needs for improved care and a new sense of a voice and empowerment. Consumerism, as a major driver of change, has only just begun. More dynamic transformational efforts are required to fully address this growing force.

## Safe Initiatives

With all the changes that have affected health care institutions in the last few decades, most fit neatly into one of five categories. Sadly, transformation at the critical core is absent in each. There is little new or innovative. That said, they are valuable and we view them as somewhat helpful initiatives in order to position an organization for more substantive and meaningful transformation efforts that still will need to be made.

**1. Improving Cost Efficiency.** As we saw at the national conference, this is what leaders are constantly seeking. Efficiency. It is characterized by realigning workflow and joining group purchasing organizations to negotiate and get concessions to get better leverage contracts for supplies and pharmaceuticals. There has been a shift from inpatient to outpatient services and facility changes and restructuring has occurred to respond to this. Many traditional providers have spent a great amount of time implementing energy savings programs, returning to in-house provided services as opposed to outsourcing and, the old standby—reducing staff.

Pursuing efficiency has been driven by an overall sense of the need to stay viable. This has always been a value of any well-run organization; but now a bunker mentality has set in. Cost efficiency is important, but it is not a panacea. It is based on a very old management model of maximizing performance through mind numbing, repetitive actions and coordination of effort to leverage size and volume of services. Major health systems still pursue this approach. We believe in efficiency, but we also believe in adaptability and identifying and implementing new behaviors or structural changes to ensure long-term sustainability. Creative and innovative change processes are put in place and enabled by strong leaders unafraid of change. A more operationally efficient organization is necessary, but not sufficient.

**2. Pay for Value.** Many traditional providers have explored, and hundreds of them have implemented, Accountable Care Organizations. These organizations were identified as a part of the Affordable Care Act and are designed to be rewarded by being accountable for improvements in care and a reduction in cost. They are paid for compliance with predetermined measures of performance. Implementation of these ACOs is in itself a major transformational change. Why? Because hospital payment for services rendered are replaced by a new financial model moving from episodic accountability to geographic, comprehensive care and population-based accountability.

The new buzzword is 'population health' and institutions are dipping their toes into this water. Certainly, payment formulas have incentivized this. Payments are based on achieving measurable quality standards and meeting patient satisfaction goals. The success sharing and bundled payments aspects built into these new models are drivers of change. It is a difficult transformation and the new models are still struggling to find their way. Current efforts at creating stronger alignments among hospitals, physicians and vendors, designed to improve care coordination, do not yet show any dramatic difference in improved patient care, financial capacity or quality scores. The promise is there. Time will tell.

3. **Disintermediation.** Increasingly, there is less and less of a need for a middleman. Internet businesses are going directly to the consumer instead of selling through a store or other setting. In health care and medical settings, disintermediation is appropriately applied to ongoing efforts to establish strong direct bonds with physicians and other providers. By exploiting new alignments and partnerships, institutions, as well as new entrants to the health care field, hope to get closer to the consumer and to provide services that are more appealing at lower cost. Brand promotion has become as ubiquitous as pharmaceutical advertising.

4. **Reducing Clinical Variation.** Evidence based medicine has been shown to improve patient outcomes. Patient safety practices have been identified and acknowledged for decades. There have been major attempts at improving quality of care and services. But, there is still too much variation in patient care found in practice behaviors, geographic regions and institutional charges. Payment formulas now consider survey scores and they measure and reward incentives for quality care and patient satisfaction. Efforts are underway to improve and to instill the best practice patterns throughout the country. It has and is going too slowly. In the preface to this book we noted studies documenting industry failure to improve and twenty years after the publication of "To Err Is Human" by the Institute of Medicine, and, in fact, no meaningful improvement in care outcomes has occurred. Researchers from the Johns Hopkins School of Medicine study on medical misbehavior reported that outcomes have slipped even more. (14) Clinical variation is the opposite of high quality.

This must be changed by the practitioners themselves. Soon. Have we fired professionals for bad clinical performance and patterns of unacceptable clinical outcomes? You bet. Did it make any long term meaningful impact on overall clinical performance? Not enough. If as many people died in any other industry as die annually from medical errors, there would be a national outcry. We consider this a safe initiative, that is uncontroversial, but it is critically important because when it comes to caring for people there is always room for improvement.

**5. Diversification**. Structural and organizational realignments have taken place in the past. But, these efforts have always been too little to make any substantive difference in the health of a patient. In many cases, they did not even contribute to the health of the institutions undergoing realignment, much less to those that they were created to serve. Some of these diversification efforts, to include institutional alignment and consolidations, have resulted in greater debt load for the larger combined organization. These alignments and new structures may be penny-wise and dollar foolish. In the short term, they may extend an organization's viability by leveraging existing contracts, payment systems and the power of increased market share. However, because debt did not decrease and fundamental changes in leadership and management did not occur; very little long-term benefit has occurred-for the patient, consumer or institution.

**Getting Unstuck**

Children are naturally very inquisitive. They are at a time in their lives when every day will present new growth. As we age, we often lose our creativity along with our questioning minds. So, it shouldn't be surprising that many organizational responses and approaches to change are risk averse, slow, uninspired and woefully lacking in substance. They are mired in the past because they can't see the forest through the trees…or, more likely, avoid even trying to look for the forest.

Traditional mindsets do not spawn creative thinking. They are stuck on the notion that if we just work faster and adjust more quickly, we will be all right. Most traditionally led organizations develop their approach for future success based on a budget as the primary driver of strategy and thus, institutional behavior is geared toward a financial goal. Future imperatives for successful health initiatives must go well beyond the traditionally developed and managed health care institution. Building a strategic plan on current operational necessities is a poor use of time and effort. It is strategically shortsighted and will eventually result in slow institutional demise. Death by a thousand cuts. We need bigger and bolder thinking in healthcare today for a more robust and impactful future.

## Keep Asking Questions

Leaders must nurture their dissatisfaction with the status quo by constantly reexamining current reality and living in a permanent state of inquiry. Strategic questions, not operational ones, must be answered before a transformational process can begin. Knowing the starting point will help immensely in charting a successful pathway on the journey. Some questions are foundational, and will help clarify where the organization is in the present. Others are more forward thinking, and will help clarify the direction the organization should best go given the new environment and the organizations purpose.

Every institution, every leader, must be able to satisfactorily function in the present while, at the same time, prepare to operate in an entirely different future environment. This is not easy to do because we cannot predict what the future will be. If we think we know what the future will be; it is almost a certainty that we will be wrong. However, we still must grasp the enormity and difficulty of strategically preparing for an unknown future. The best way to do this is to reorient our thought processes from a centric-based organizational perspective to an outside environmental model. It is thinking from the outside in.

## Outside-In Thinking

Traditionally established and managed health care institutions have old approaches to planning for the future. They tend to ask, "What do we want to be, where do we need to go, and, how much money do we need to generate? This is an inside-out orientation. The organization is the epicenter. It is driven by pressure from physicians, bondholders and historical perspectives. The path forward is whatever the organization deems it should be to achieve its own internally generated definition of success.

A different orientation has greater and longer-term sustainable advantage. It is a more open-minded way of viewing potentially transformative events outside of ourselves. It can have a profound and significant influence on the purpose and function of the organization. It is not for the faint of heart. Outside-In Thinking challenges organizations and leaders to look at a larger world to assess the impact of major events, drivers of change and developing environmental dynamics on the world in which we work and live. There are social, technical, political, environmental and economic drivers of change that are bigger than any one organization. It is best to try to understand the major waves of change that will sweep all in the same direction. No organization is immune to the changes that will come.

Ignoring outside forces ensures that an organization's future will be shaped by such forces. When the wave of change finally crashes on the shore, they are caught off guard and will not be able to withstand its energy. Being prepared for major transformational events brings clarity to honestly confront potential scenarios. Some scenarios may be scary and far-fetched, but by being open, a bold new future can be envisioned and then pursued with confidence and foresight.

We borrowed the concept of *outside-in thinking* from Shell Oil company as it was described in The Art of the Long View by Peter Schwarz. (15) It has been also used by others in healthcare. Outside-In Thinking involves understanding very large and significant movements in the world, i.e., events over which one has absolutely no control, but which could have a significant impact on organizational performance, and even survival. This approach recognizes and does not overlook things that are a bit closer to home; like: market share, volatility, consumer demands and needs, competitors, vendors and typical institutional assessments of internal strengths and weaknesses. These are the areas often identified by most organizations as the basis for their long-range strategic planning. In our view, basing a plan solely on near-term implications of competitive position and present-day challenges and circumstances is simply not sufficient for any sort of meaningful long term transformational consideration. Especially in the health care world. The concept of thinking from the outside-in instead of the inside-out is offers a better way of viewing, preparing for, and achieving success from long term implications and opportunities.

**No Mission Impossible**

**A mission statement is the most important aspect of an organization's strategic approach to the future.** All organizations should have one. It is the foundational piece upon which everything else is built. It is used in branding and marketing materials. Its community, employees and consumers know what it means.

The strategic plan and tactics are set in motion to build and support the mission, rather than to achieve a predetermined financial goal or other short-term yardsticks. While a mission-driven organization's character is well grounded, its course is adaptable in the face of evolving environmental realities.

A clue to determining if the mission statement is understood is to look carefully at the practice of the people in the workplace. Their behaviors should reflect intent. Do the doctors, staff, board and other professionals behave in alignment with the meaning of the purpose statement? Do rewards or incentives line up with the intent of the mission's words? Are job descriptions reflecting the purpose of the institution, or are they outdated? Does the unspoken intent of the organization mirror the true intent of the organization?

**Once the mission of the organization is understood and accepted as the most import driver, ask: Is your core business the right business for the future?** Are you even in the right business? For example, the Benedictine Sisters of Boerne, Texas determined that operating their small hospitals was not serving people as well as they thought they should be served. They also concluded that, given their relative size and the economic viability of the markets they served, they would not last long in their present organizational paradigm. So, in line with their mission, they made a bold move. In the mid-1980s they sold their healthcare facilities and funded new initiatives in advocacy and social responsibility. With carefully researched and well articulated policy positions they have since served millions of people by advocating to change systemic issues, obstacles and state law in order to improve healthcare. They have magnified the impact of their service and commitment well beyond what it would have been if they had only continued in hospital operations.

There comes a time when the forms and formulas must change. The way that healthcare is currently delivered is not sustainable in the long term. In tough times, it is tempting to 'hunker down.' However, it is even more important for healthcare leaders to reiterate the higher purpose of their calling. Significant and meaningful goals that benefit all who are to be served should be identified and emphasized. Doing so may confront an organization's current reality. This is the edge of change. Steps need to be taken. Questions need to be asked and tough challenges addressed.

**The Market Need**

**WHO will need to be served in 10 or 20 years?**

This question can be easily addressed by measuring the impact of demography. Demographic knowledge tells us about the expected size and age of a population. It can tell us the extent of diversity and differences in makeup of the population. It can even forecast characteristics of future generations.

But, numbers aren't everything. Quantitative numbers do not tell us the needs, desires, wants or conditions determined by economic and social values. Anticipatory and effective leaders must identify potential gaps in services, and understand the difference between the haves and the have-nots of the future generation. Health care institutions must remain engaged in their communities.

**HOW should we serve people 10 or 20 years from now?**

Looking back, it is easy to see how much has changed in a short period of time. Technological advances were major contributors. While we can't predict all technological advances, we can reliably say that the speed of technological change is accelerating. Therefore, we can presume that clinical, medical and technical advances will be on a lightning track. These technological changes have an influence on our lives, our social infrastructure and our communication. They reset expectations of performance and satisfactory outcomes.

Here is how we might answer this question:

- The current trend of migrating services out of the acute care hospital to other settings will continue. Home will be a growing and more common site for care and service delivery.
- The local pharmacy will become more important to consumers than the doctor's office. It might even replace the doctor's office for the majority of primary care.
- The role of physicians will change over time. They will be less independent and become more of a team and a partner, joining other physicians or physician extenders to serve patients more holistically.
- The evolution of medical school curriculum will include more emphasis on community and population health. Medical schools will teach students to rely on the team more than on themselves.

Given the changes that we know will occur, and accepting that there will be other, unforeseen, powerful influences, scenario planning, a key component of outside-in thinking, is an important tool to prepare on organization for the many future possibilities. This important tool is discussed later in this book.

**WHAT will be the expectations of the healthcare consumer 10 or 20 years from now, and how do we live up to them?**

The consumer will expect a higher level of performance, access, communication, transparency, accuracy, and speed. All that, for less money.

To be relevant in the next decade and beyond, engaged organizations must develop a deep understanding of consumers' expectations and plan for a more consumer-centric world. The old definition of health, which has come from an over reliance on professional educators, statistics and data does not speak to the new generation of health consumer.

The trend is for people to place a greater emphasis on spirituality and an integrated approach to being well. Emotional and mental health will continue to gain great traction in the minds of people. Integrative medicine is an orientation that is expanding what it means to be a health care provider. Employers are also reexamining what it means to have a 'healthy workforce' and their part in making this possible.

What will have to be different about your organization to be responsive to new demands? Becoming a true participant (not just the large organizational presence) within social, religious and community networks is vital for engagement and community acceptance. Continued investment in bricks and mortar must be re-considered. What was once the symbol of a successful medical care institution, its large buildings and campus, will likely become future burdens. This likelihood is particularly true for institutions that are currently operating on 'the margins'.

The best investment for your institution, and for the community, will be human resources. Young leaders must be identified, groomed and taught how to manage accelerating change, creative out-of-the-box and outside-in thinking and the techniques of future thinking. The all-knowing, wise and charismatic leader of best selling books is passé. New leadership must be focused and anticipatory, diverse and holders of broad experience, perspectives and skills. They must be courageous without being egocentric. Leaders must be willing to abandon the past, and pursue the road less traveled. They must create settings in which their co-collaborators/employees can find and add value to society.

Entrepreneurial mindsets and winning approaches to serving the greater good in new ways must be rewarded and fostered. Many clinicians have more to offer than technical skills. They have the background and personal style that enable them to serve in leadership roles. They should be identified, encouraged, and assisted to do so.

Rethink the model of care delivery. Assess what is best in your community by being a good listener and a community partner. Establish new metrics for success. Allocate ample time, money and human resources. Pilot test the new model while maintaining existing services. If warranted, move to a new way of serving. The challenge is to provide new knowledge for others to use in innovative strategic ways. Don't put new wine in old wineskins. Make sure the structure is redone to hold the new model in order to ensure its success.

## WHAT are the broader community needs?

In the past, we often defined community need based on what we had to give to the community because it was accretive to the institution. If we were a cancer hospital, then surely there must be a community need for cancer screening and follow-up therapies. Taking a step back, we should ask if we truly offer services that meet community needs, or are we just providing the ones for which we get paid?

A community and its health service providers are mutually dependent on each other. The broader community requires access to a healthcare provider. Good healthcare ensures economic vitality, employment opportunities and health security for its citizens. Obviously, a hospital cannot exist without a community. It provides a service in time of crisis and, now more often than not, it provides health care services to the chronically ill of a community. Such mutual interdependence, as opposed to mutual exploitation, is beneficial to all parties. The concept of a 'social contract" between those with services and those in need of services exists and must be understood. It is important to collaboratively, constantly and comprehensively be in a positive and engaged relationship with the community. It can be tempting to 'stick to ones knitting,' to focus on the demands of the institution and let the outside world alone. It is easier. But, this is short sighted and is a pathway to breaking the social contract.

A core strategy for long-term viability is to identify partnerships and collaborative approaches with key constituents well beyond the traditional quasi partners of the past. One must be a good listener to be a good partner, one must be humble, walk the path, and have shared experiences to build trust. Stay engaged in constant dialogue to foster a partnership that raises all boats. Health care is too complicated and complex to walk alone.

**HOW can you be a vital contributor in the future environment?**

Strategic thinking is challenging. It is not one-dimensional. It is not even two-dimensional. It requires a multidimensional perspective.

A leader cannot determine where to go without having a thorough understanding and knowledge of where the institution is and was. This is a foundational aspect of establishing strategic direction. It is the springboard from which to go forward. Understanding the past is to understand history, in the context of institutional intentions. But knowledge does not make identifying the best path forward any easier. It has been said that the past is the best predictor of the future. Not anymore.

There are so many variables that go into developing a sound strategy. Strategy, effectively developed, is hard work. Sadly, many very competent people will not put in the time and energy to do it well. A solid strategic plan cannot be developed over an extended lunch. For the health care industry, upon which whole communities lean for economic and physical well-being, there is a need for big, broad, outside-in thinking.

**The Finish Line**

Implementing a successful transformation is time consuming, and requires constant vigilance and effort. It can also be energizing, affirming and beneficial. While there will be dustups along the way, there should be even more celebrations at the finish line.

A successful transformational effort must be grounded in culture. This takes time. Stick with it. Hold people accountable. Reward them. Celebrate successes. At the end of the day, if the organization continues, or better yet enhances and improves, how it serves its community and becomes a stronger and more dynamic entity, then you will know your transformational efforts have been successful.

# Chapter 2

# The Barriers to Transformational Change

**"Knowing is not enough; we must apply.**
**Willing is not enough; we must do." - Goethe**

## Knowing Is Not Enough; Implementation Is Key

No one is perfect, but we expect perfection in our health care practitioner and facility. Those at the helm of health care organizations are very talented, bright people. But, they are human, and mistakes don't escape them, nor anyone else within the medical community. That's one of the reasons why the management of all facets relating to health care needs to be done with a keen eye, kid gloves, and plenty of quality controls.

The latest technology and finest equipment don't always equate to quality health care. In fact, in a recent U.S. Senate hearing, physicians from Harvard, confirmed that hospitals were no safer than they were 15 years' prior (16) when the Institute of Medicine report "Is Human" drew national concern and attention.

Over the last 25 years, much has been written about strategies to improve the quality and costs of health care in the United States. Using new and more sophisticated data analysis, some hospitals and health systems have designed what appear to be stronger road maps to address the significant challenges they face today. Those prospering institutions have excellent quality indicators, patient satisfaction, physician performance exceeding the norm and sound financial practices leading to solid and balanced outcomes.

Yet, many others have made little or no efforts to implement successful transformational strategies or focus on quality and safety outcome measures. In the end, there are significantly more organizations posting negative results, thereby canceling the positive gains.

What could be the reasons for this lack of progress, particularly in light of the availability of knowledgeable solutions? The answer is clear. *Just knowing the road map to the future is not enough.* Organizational transformation that achieves positive results in patient care, satisfaction and outcomes *requires implementation of the strategies* that drive the journey of improvement in all aspects of the organization. This can be painful. Short term financial hits can and will occur. Disorientation and confusion are a certainty. Overcoming lethargy and inaction are the toughest obstacles of all.

**Barriers to Implementation**

Successful implementation of any plan can be complex and challenging, especially one that drives significant organizational transformation. Undoubtedly, leaders oftentimes face significant barriers preventing them from achieving their goals. These barriers must be understood and eventually overcome in order to get from point A to point B. Potential barriers can fit into five categories.

**One: Lack of Urgency to Change**

Change under many conditions is difficult and painful for some people. This difficulty manifests itself in several barriers that blind them to the urgency for change.

- Comfort with the Status Quo. Being uncomfortable with the present situation is necessary to urge people to make changes.

Change requires energy, focus, elimination or major modification of once-successful behaviors, strategies and tactics. That's a tall order, so some leaders develop a high level of comfort with the status quo. These individuals become the resistors of change. They are often immobilized by the fear of walking into new territory, being unsure of what they may find. This fear, if not overcome, makes staying where they are the only option.

- <u>Unable to Recognize When the Platform Is Burning</u>. A commonly used term in business lexicon is the "burning platform". The term refers to the need for a dramatic and drastic change (or choice) because the existing situation has finally become untenable...a burning platform. Some underperforming facilities are closing, and better-performing organizations acquire others. Layoffs and downsizing are the norm. Physician relationships continue to be stressful and complicated because of various employment and contract arrangements. Balance sheets are deteriorating, and days-in-cash are declining. Revenue enhancement becomes extremely difficult. All bond-rating agencies warn of a negative outlook for the health care sector. Despite knowing and seeing this happen around them, some leaders still convince themselves the need for change is not urgent. They either believe the platform is not burning, or if it is, it is not hot enough.

- <u>Unwilling to Face the Toxic Side Effects</u>. Road maps aren't always easy going down a super highway. Likewise, in health care management, where treatments must be modified based on new knowledge, and processes and procedures must be redesigned for successful transformation, toxic side effects will occur. Although they are expected and interpreted by many as negative, they are positive evidence that change has been implemented. An example of an undesirable side effect in the clinical setting is hair loss experienced by cancer patients undergoing chemotherapy. After weeks of treatment, the physician does not ask the bald patient, "Oh, no, what have we done?" The doctor recognizes hair loss as a positive, but toxic, side effect. Hence, the physician says, "Good. The treatment is working." Some leaders cannot apply the same logic to the clinical and administrative changes needed to made each day in order to achieve excellence. So, when they see the toxic side effects of change, they see them as negatives and then convince themselves that change is not worth the accompanying short-term toxicity.

## Two: Financial Barriers

Transformational success requires significant changes in all aspects of health care, including the approach to financial and business literacy. Any organization's journey into the future must be driven by a sound business plan, and supported by sustainable financial outcomes. Just as sound financial principles are essential in the future, current financial processes in the industry create barriers to moving forward.

- Money. One of the root causes of the health care crisis, and its resistance to any normal corrective action, has and will continue to be the historical flow of money into the industry. Leaders have been reluctant to implement transformational plans because there have been no economic reasons to change… until recently. Yes, there have been some economic blips, and casualties, along the way. But for every minor mishap, a newer, stronger organization has arrived on the scene to take advantage of the economic opportunities. Metaphorically, health care has proven to be an unending economic gold rush of undetermined potential. There are many who believe there are no signs of the mother lode running out. We have had personal conversations with senior leaders who, still today, expect the gold rush to continue to produce at historical or even higher levels. It is extremely difficult to convince someone with this mind-set to change. Hence one more reason, and perhaps the most important reason, current health care leaders are so averse to change.

- Insulation from Economic Realities. The health care industry has been insulated from economic and normal business realities because of governmental programs, insurers' profitability, employers' willingness to cover their employees' health care costs, physicians who have been able to increase their incomes every year, and the successful advocacy programs of medical and administrative associations. Patients do not know the true costs of their procedures, treatments and medications because their insurance coverage protects them from it. Governmental programs and regulations have, in many cases, restricted real, unvarnished knowledge about the largest industry in the United States.

- Lack of Financial Resources. Leaders readily accept that, "When you are out of cash, you are out of luck." Today, the strength of balance sheets and days in cash would indicate some health care entities are on their way to failure. Yes, many transformational strategies require money. For example, money is helpful to renovate unused real estate, to recruit competent leaders and physicians to develop new services, and for staff professional development to learn how to effectively implement the road map to success. Leaders with limited resources, perhaps pondering how they will make the next payroll, are likely to stand in place rather than move forward.

**Three: Not Recognizing the New Rebar**

Clayton Christensen, in his book, <u>The Innovators Dilemma</u> about business disruption- as is occurring in health care today, used the steel industry as an example of positive transformation. (17) When those making steel faced significant challenges in the 1980s, some of the failing companies were determined to survive, to change and to succeed. They retooled, transforming their operations to make rebar. Doing so, they represented change occurring in the market. These survivors embraced new technologies, cost-structure advantages, and new business models. Companies that did not transform, if they stayed in the steel business, went bankrupt or closed. They did not recognize the need to make changes to survive and flourish in changing and dynamic markets.

This lack of recognition creates numerous barriers to change today. No matter what business one can think of there will always be **New Entrants in the Market.** One need not travel far to see freestanding urgent-care centers, emergency rooms and walk-in clinics rising out of the ground. Doctor-owned hospitals, which do not rely on governmental payments, are increasing, as are ambulatory surgery centers where physicians are the major partners. Within large pharmacy chains and department stores, full-service, primary-care clinics, staffed by nurse practitioners, are springing up. A new construct, a hospital without beds, is now in operation using only advanced telecommunications equipment to maintain contact with and provide services to patients. With just a few locations, Cancer Centers of America, advertise that they are a national system equipped with the latest technologies, and can provide you with an appointment today. These new entrants in the market create solutions traditional delivery systems have missed.

Particularly in healthcare, the **Growth of Non-Physician Providers** looms as a major innovation. Given the lack of primary-care physicians, many states have significantly increased the scope of responsibilities for nurse practitioners and physician assistants, including writing prescriptions. Contrary to what some physicians think, the research on these nurses' practices indicates outcomes are equally as good, or better, then physicians for a large set of diagnoses. They often have significantly higher patient-satisfaction scores also.

We consider a subset of the non-traditional approach to healthcare to be **Alternative or Complementary Medicine Becoming Mainstream**. As patients find success and satisfaction with such modalities as acupuncture, herbal medicine and other therapies, there is a reduction in frequency of visits to allopathic practitioners. Additionally, 50 percent of health care consumption is self-prescribed through the purchase of vitamins, over-the-counter medications, natural supplements and other things. (18)

The **Role of the Government and Employers** is evolving and changing rapidly. Today's reality is that both governmental programs and employer-based insurance, because of their unsustainable costs, are aggressively focused on reducing the rate of growth of the increase in reimbursement health care from their historical levels. In 2010, the government made its statement about the future of care through the passage of the Affordable

Care Act (ACA). The government is now revisiting the ACA but will continue to make a statement about healthcare delivery. Multiple companies have gone through bankruptcy to reduce what they would have had to pay in health care costs. Some companies have even closed plants or moved from a location after failing to reduce their health care costs to an acceptable level. (19) Companies are now willing to take the necessary steps to get workers to accept the benefit changes required to create a sustainable and stable business model.

Another role that is changing is that of the **Payers**. Although third-party payers have been a key component of what has driven health care in the United States to where it is today, they are now recognizing that change (read reducing) in their payment for care and service is critical to survival. Insurance companies are also beginning to experience margin compression as the ACA is adding more individuals to insurance rolls who cannot pay even the reduced premiums. This is driving payers to design and require the adoption of narrow networks for services for the patient. The payers will continue to do what is necessary to reduce their costs and preserve their margins.

### Four: Ineffective Leadership and Governance

Successful transformation will not occur unless the CEO, leadership team, and the board of trustees perform effectively at all times. Rather than encouraging transformation, many C-suite executives and board members become barriers to success. All leaders and trustees must have a set of competencies to drive positive outcomes with regard to operations, strategic directions and generative thinking. Sadly, in today's dynamic environment the competencies that got leaders into the positions that they now occupy are not sufficient for tomorrow. They need to collaborate instead of compete. Being collaborative, rather than competitive, is critical. This holds true for internal team members, providers and even what was once considered competition. We are all human beings and so we must recognize that ego and arrogance are a part of the human condition, but they are deadly. Because of the complexity of the challenges in health care today, the design of the solutions will take the brainpower and robust dialogue of many. This group effort is weakened if the voice of one is always louder than the others. Ego can destroy the collective energy and forward momentum of the group. Arrogance often leads senior people to ignore data and rely on their instinct instead of facts, on their experience instead of knowledge. Arrogance has led to monuments that now stand half full. There are bed towers being built that will, eventually, stand completely empty because of the expectation that volumes of people are waiting to enter the hospital door. "If we can just expand the building..." is no longer a sound strategy. Unveiling new operating rooms will not always assure more surgeries. This may be the case in markets with a younger population, where trauma is high, or where income levels are increasing. However, these community characteristics are not the norm. It is our opinion that only in an organically growing community with an economically advantaged population can an assessment conclude that growth of facility services is reasonable. This can foster the belief that more is better. This, in turn, can drive an ill-advised plan to lead an organization on an unsustainable path. Be careful what you wish for. Leave your ego at home. Challenge your beliefs.

**Five: Ignoring Best Practices**

Although health care leaders are working today in the most challenging environment ever experienced, they usually can find a proven best practice. These practices, whether they are clinical, administrative or technological, can be transported back into their own organization with little or no tweaking. By not looking externally for solutions, leaders are ignoring pathways for success. We have found patterns that undermine potential. Pay attention to these common pitfalls:

- Not Utilizing Evidenced-Based Data and Research. If you are thinking about doing something new, there is probably someone, somewhere who has figured out how to do it right already. The Internet provides immediate access to a wealth of such knowledge. Keeping a catalogue of internal best practices is also critical, particularly in large systems where the right hand often does not know what the left hand is doing. If there are barriers to such

27

sharing practices, much waste will occur of the team's time and organizational resources.

- Not Embracing Clinical Technologies. Clinical technology must be embraced to help drive organizational change. The rapid development and implementation of new, less invasive, safer, and often more cost effective clinical technologies has resulted in decreasing hospital admissions, better outcomes and shorter recovery periods. Such is evidenced in the five-minute cataract surgery and 30-minute gall bladder removal, commonly done in outpatient facilities. We hear leaders, including physicians, pining for the "good old days." When you really study those days, you will often find the only thing good was the revenue generated by long lengths of stays for the hospital and concurrent daily care charges for the physicians.

- Not Supporting Information Technology. There is no room for error in the decision-making processes for leadership and the trustees. There is no money to squander. Poor information results in wasted energy for leaders, and minimizes their ability to successfully address the highest priorities for change. The best decisions are informed decisions, utilizing every ounce of data available. This requires cutting-edge information technology, capable of analyzing the data in a meaningful way for the decision makers.

- A Non-Innovative Environment. Innovative thinking results in innovative changes, which help to drive an organization forward. These changes may be responsible for a hospital or system maintaining its position, or claiming the lead in the market. A non-innovative environment fosters a path that slows or even stifles the transformational process.

## Six: Tolerance of Mediocrity

The tolerance of mediocrity is one of the greatest barriers to achieving meaningful improvements on a continuing journey to excellence. If the tolerance of mediocrity is prevalent and visible, it will frustrate many high performers as they realize that outstanding work is not valued in the organization. Consequently, a portion of the high achievers may slip and become slackers. As mediocrity takes over, the chances of achieving excellence in the company are significantly compromised. To illustrate, when one of the authors, Dr. Tom was responsible for all clinicians at the Geisinger Clinic, he had to address mediocrity and eliminate it as he would a cancer. In one instance a surgeon, a former college football player who was a strong, intimidating person and who had failed numerous attempts at corrective action regarding his mediocre performance, had to be called into Dr. Tom's office for a final decision. A letter of resignation was written for the surgeon to sign so that he could be discharged from the Geisinger Clinic. This was handed to the surgeon who promptly told Dr. Tom that he could take that letter and shove it up his butt; and, as he did this, he lifted the chair in which was sitting as if to throw it. Dr. Tom responded, "In that case I am going to need two copies of this letter". The surgeon began to laugh, signed the letter and left the organization. Tolerance of mediocrity cannot be condoned, but we must always retain our humanity and humor and, if we do, the good and right thing will result.

In summary, the barriers for transformational implementation are numerous, and provide what some leaders and physicians believe are good reasons for not changing. No reason is acceptable. If we do not change, we will continue to have a delivery system with high cost and low quality, questionable safety and poor patient outcomes. Most important, by benignly supporting an environment that allows unacceptable outcomes, we are violating the sacred trust that patients and their families have in health care providers when they turn over their most important gift — their lives. Surely this demands that the blinders must come off, barriers must be eliminated, and the drivers of change must be identified and heeded. The future must be imagined and envisioned. Strong leaders must do what is necessary and right, and implement it.

# Chapter 3

# The Drivers of
# Transformational Change

**"Change or Die" -- Alan Deutschman**

What drives transformational change? By simple definition, transformation means becoming something different. A common example in nature is a caterpillar transforming into a butterfly. Based on our research within health care industry and other industries, we have identified three primary drivers that stimulate transformation; and existential crisis, a leader with a compelling vision, and the innate human need to succeed.

**Organizational Crisis**. In Chapter Two we referred to this as the burning platform. This is not the normal, garden-variety challenging issues that all organizations face at one time or another. Instead these are negative circumstances that put the future of an organization in jeopardy. This can manifest as organizational chaos that oftentimes results in CEO termination. Organizational crisis might be felt as entering survival mode. When the threats facing the organization are so significant, improvement initiatives are no longer an adequate response. Dramatic transformation is required to survive.

**Visionary Leadership**. Sometimes it's an individual, and other times it's the collective vision of several individuals that stimulate an organization to positive change. These people are legendary, and their biographies abound. In many instances, these visionaries created industries, or revolutionized existing industries. Their legacies are reflected in the enterprises they founded or turned around. Through their vision, they saw and created a very different organization that was poised to succeed in the future.

**Entrepreneurship**. Especially in a capitalistic and competitive business ecosystem, entrepreneurs seeking economic opportunity drive transformational change. To ignore recent history in the world of IPOs and acquisitions would be a significant oversight in what drives transformational change. Microsoft and Apple are almost graybeards when thinking about technology companies. Facebook, YouTube, LinkedIn, Instagram, Tumblr, Nest, WhatsApp, Autonomy, and Beats are just a few examples of companies that have transformed their founders into billionaires.

## The Genesis of Transformation

In the book, <u>Only the Paranoid Survive</u>, Andrew Grove (20) describes how he and Gordon Moore, Intel's chairman and chief executive officer, were confronted with the potential failure of the company because of the changing marketplace from memory chips to microprocessors. During this period, Grove recounts how they were confronted with the issue. "If we got kicked out, and the board brought in a new CEO, what do you think he would do?" Their answer was to get out of memory chips and into microprocessors. With this decision, they changed the course of Intel. Transformation, however, is not an instantaneous process. It took Intel three years to transform from one business to another. Launching a transformational journey within an industry-leading incumbent organization before a major crisis occurs is very difficult. Most leaders wait too long to launch this type of transformational initiative. Intel's Andrew Grove and Gordon Moore became legendary transformational leaders because they called the question on themselves.

Apple is another excellent example of transformative change of two varieties. Founded by Steve Jobs and Steve Wozniak in 1976, Apple was one of the transformative companies credited with launching the personal computer industry. (21) This is the type of transformational journey stimulated by visionary individuals. Over the course of the next 20 years, Apple would decline to almost the point of bankruptcy. With the financial condition of Apple in serious turmoil, Steve Jobs returned and created a second transformation. Using the environment of operational chaos and organizational distress, Jobs created a vision for a new Apple around music, books, photographs, and videos with creations like iTunes, the iPod, the iPhone, the iMac, and the iPad. Many consider the magnitude of the second transformation even greater than the original formation of the company. The transformed Apple emerged with a market capitalization of more than $700 billion.

Intel and Apple represent two very high-profile technology transformation stories. Health care has had similar high-profile transformational organizations. Started in 1962 with their first nursing home, David A. Jones Sr. and H. Wendell Cherry formed what would become the largest nursing home operation in the United States by 1969. In the 1980s, Jones and Cherry left long-term care and transformed their business into one of the largest publicly traded, multi-hospital systems in the United States: Humana. In the 1990s, the company was split into Humana insurance, and a hospital company that was subsequently sold to HCA. In 2015, Humana began another transformation from "managing risk" to "improving clinical outcomes." So, over the course of 40 years, Humana has undergone numerous transformations. (22)

Another transformational health care example is the Geisinger Health System. In 1915, Abigail Geisinger, along with Harold Foss, MD, formed the George F. Geisinger Memorial Hospital in Danville, Pennsylvania. Prior to coming to Danville, Dr. Foss spent a 20-month fellowship as an assistant to Dr. William Mayo at the Mayo Clinic in Rochester, Minnesota. Dr. Foss transported the Mayo model of employed physicians to the Geisinger Hospital. In addition, Dr. Foss initiated, for the first time in the United States, paid internships and residences in internal medicine, cardiology and general surgery. This organizational structure, along with the physician residencies, would become one of the first of its kind in the United States. In 1985, Geisinger would transform itself by adding a health-maintenance organization, the Geisinger Health Plan. This would make the organization one of the first fully integrated health care delivery systems that included physicians, a hospital and an insurance company all under a single operating umbrella. In 2005, the Geisinger Board asked leadership to increase innovation around chronic care and illness prevention. This would become Geisinger ProvenCare. Under this transformational model, Geisinger provides guaranteed price and outcome for selected services. This has become one of the prototypes for the value-based payment models under development by the Centers for Medicare and Medicaid Services. (23)

While health care has, and must continue to have, major transformation to succeed, perhaps no other industry has undergone as much transformation as the airline industry. At least one location for the beginning of this transformation was Texas. In 1971, Southwest Airlines started as a regional airline operating between Dallas, San Antonio and Houston. The transformational business model was to be a low-cost travel provider to people that typically would drive, travel by train, or ride the bus. Short trips (500 miles), one type of aircraft (Boeing 737), rapid turnaround of planes on the ground (20 minutes), no assigned seats, no meal service, no external reservation system, no baggage transfer between different airlines, being fun to fly, and general frugality were the critical factors to meeting the business strategy. An objective of the Southwest founders was to democratize airline travel for everyone. Almost half a century later, the airline industry has been revolutionized by many of the business strategies Southwest Airlines introduced. (24)

The purpose of sharing these stories is to illustrate how transformation can occur anywhere and in any industry. The genesis of a transformational thought can also originate from anywhere. The result of transformation can have devastating effects on business incumbents. The survival of incumbents isn't very high in transformed industries. At Intel, incumbent leaders posed to themselves a very challenging "what if" question regarding the future of the organization. At Apple, founding leaders departed the organization, and over time, the personal computer industry that the company helped invent left them behind as other manufacturers commoditized the hardware. As health care developed from a relatively inconsequential cottage industry into a $3 trillion juggernaut, many stories of transformation can be found. No industry is completely insulated from factors that generate transformational interventions.

These examples illustrate how transformation goes far beyond improvement. Business literature contains many books about operational improvement. Numerous concepts have been developed to further operational improvement. Business reengineering, total quality management (TQM), continuous process improvement (CPI), lean manufacturing, Six Sigma, supply chain management, management by objective (MBO), key performance indicators (KPIs), balanced scorecards, and benchmarking are just a few of the many theories developed, over the past 40 years, to improve business performance. The drivers of the need for operational improvement are always self-evident. For example, organizational performance is declining; higher-quality and lower-cost producers enter the market and capture market share; new technology provides competitors with advantages; changes in customer expectations; or Wall Street demands. Benchmarking creates operational improvement. Customer satisfaction surveys create operational improvement. These factors are important to any business, but they aren't the drivers behind transformational change.

Transformational change originates from a different place than process improvement efforts. Memory chips aren't microprocessors. The personal computer isn't an iPhone, iPod or iPad. A hospital employing physicians and operating an insurance company is very different from a standalone hospital. Nursing homes' services are far from those provided at acute care hospitals, and the insurance industry is much different from either of those. For consumers, who don't typically drive transformation, the differences may not be understandable because of technical nuances. However, consumers benefit from the visions and passions of transformational leaders who see the world differently, and make a difference in the status quo.

## Ingredients for Transformation

If you have an organizational crisis, a vision for a uniquely different future, or an entrepreneurial spirit, you have the necessary ingredients to launch your own transformational journey. There is also a set of enablers that, along with these drivers, can facilitate the journey.

**The ability to communicate** the vision with others, and build a team, is an important enabler. This is where the obstacles immediately become more challenging. Organizational culture and existing business inertia can be insurmountable obstacles to transformative change. Behavioral psychology, cognitive science and neuroscience have recently provided great insights as to how associates adapt to change. Alan Deutschman, in his book "Change or Die," presents the case that 90 percent of people having coronary-artery bypass surgery are unable to change their lifestyles to prevent future cardiac events that possibly could kill them. (25) Transformational change within existing organizations is equally difficult.

Similarly, leaders within organizations with followers unwilling to join in the process face a monumental obstacle to overcome to create transformational change. Communicating and selling a compelling vision of the future to enlist the hearts and minds of an organization's workforce is a most difficult task that any leader faces. Ultimately, no transformational change occurs without teamwork. Very seldom is ultimate transformational change the result of a single individual. In studying transformational companies, one will find partners, small groups, like-minded colleagues, collaborators, or advocates at ground zero. Many of these names are icons: Steve Jobs, Steve Wozniak and Mike Markkula at Apple; Rollin King, Herb Kelleher, John Peace, Colleen Barrett, and Lamar Muse at Southwest Airlines; Abigail Geisinger and Dr. Harold Foss at Geisinger; David A. Jones Sr. and H. Wendell Cherry at Humana.

**Know-how** is another critical enabler. A level of competence to bring about the transformation is necessary. Products or services must ultimately find customers. Being able to build, implement, and execute the new concept is critical to success. The challenge associated with this enabler is finding team members that are willing to let go of the past, and not attempt to drag it into the future. Finding the people who have the adaptability to understand the constraints of the status quo, but not be inhibited by them, is critical. Historically, this is the example used over and over of how incumbent companies were unable to see the future that someone else did, despite being in the business. Motorola succumbed to the smartphone. Braniff, Northwest, Republic, Frontier, and Eastern were just a few of the many airline companies that were merged, bought or discontinued because of the change in competition. Sony was in both the technology and music businesses but didn't see the iPod opportunity. Disruptive paradigm shifts are alive and well.

Finally, the intangibles—**self-confidence, energy, enthusiasm, tenacity, passion, inspiration, and motivation**—are all enablers of transformational change. The gravitational pull of the status quo is extremely powerful. The ease of diligently working to improve the known is much less stressful than attempting to invent something brand-new. Convincing investors, boards and others of the need for transformational change can be challenging. Selling an unknown future can be very difficult. The risk of loss by incumbents in tangential businesses creates immediate competitive reactions.

Two health care organizations, Geisinger and Humana, were earlier presented as transformative organizations. Future organizational transformation in health care will be extremely difficult. Industry momentum, societal expectations, incumbent oligopolies, government regulations, policy makers, financial incentives, and industry size make organizational transformation beyond challenging in health care. During the financial crisis of 2007, we became familiar with the terminology "too big to fail." This descriptor was used to describe organizations that were deemed too large to be allowed to go bankrupt because of the greater risk their failure might inflict on the entire financial system. As an industry, health care includes many incumbent organizations that during a time of transformational upheaval could attain this same critical status.

With the baby boomers ready for Medicare, policy makers and politicians will be constrained by the imagined or real backlash from any potential disruption of the health care benefits provided by this program. On the other side of the coin, the continued increase in health care costs creates the potential of the program collapsing under its own financial weight. In theory, this type of economic condition would be the perfect trigger to set in motion transformational change. The past financial crisis, however, might indicate that economic conditions have not deteriorated far enough to create the necessary anxiety to overcome the current inertia of the status quo. The storm is formed and approaching. Woe to those who are unprepared.

# Chapter 4

# The Future Health Care Landscape

**"Use What You Have. Do What You Can." -- Arthur Ashe**

Once the drivers of the significant changes transforming the health care landscape are understood and the barriers to implementing the change strategies and tactics are overcome, or at least minimized, the organization's transformational journey can begin. If this journey is to be successful, it is necessary for leaders to envision the future health care landscape into which the organization must travel and where it must not only survive, but thrive.

Getting to this new destination will not be easy. Change journeys are seen by many as extremely difficult, and create much anxiety and fear in travelers who prefer the status quo. Future success depends on the recognition by the board, the CEO, the leadership team, the physicians, and the management teams that change is critical for survival and will be a constant for the long-term future. Hopefully, most will find the journey into the future health care landscape not only a challenging opportunity but also an exciting and energizing one.

## Components of the Future Landscape

The myriad changes creating the future health care landscape can best be understood and addressed if they are categorized under six key areas.

The future landscape will demand new areas of focus.

## Rethinking the Clinicians Role

- Value versus Volume. In the past, volume was a primary driver for revenue. Just as in any industry, when the focus is on volume, quality is harder to control. In the health care arena, we saw that high volume led to extreme variability in outcomes. Overuse and misuse of treatment modalities were rampant. In the changing landscape, providers will be paid for what is "best" rather than what is "more."

- Health and Wellness. More focus will be on preventing diseases. This growing emphasis on wellness will result in many strategies and tactics to grow well care, hence reducing the need for sick care.

- Patient Centricity. For decades, U.S. health care has been designed around what works best for the provider. This notion is a little understood by consumers, but in fact, the premise has been that providers represent the patient and therefore everything they do must certainly have the patients interests at heart. If this were true, physicians would still be making house calls. In today's customer-centric environment, we need to turn that old blueprint around. In other words, a transformation of delivery processes is essential.

- Meeting the Needs of the Community. Health care is a community asset. This will never change. Consequently, driving transformation based on needs that are identified through a current community health assessment will be required. When we were running our last organization, we mandated that community needs assessments were to be written by the community and not by us. Of course, we were part of the process, we were the conveners, but our primary purpose was to listen openly and be prepared to respond honestly. Many times, our resources were not prepared to meet the needs of the community as the members of the community had defined them. But, it was our obligation to help to enable these needs to be met, which often required us to start new programs, to collaborate with other providers and to fund initiatives through grants that, in fact, had no direct connection to any of our services or programs.

- <u>Evidenced-Based Medicine</u>. Utilizing the best clinical practices proven by evidence gained through research will be significantly more consequential as value overtakes volume.

## The Changing Face of Disease

Just as smallpox has been eradicated and numerous childhood cancers are maintained in permanent remission, so too will some additional diseases be added to the "cured" list as the transformation landscape unfolds. Identifying those that will disappear from the need for future service must be anticipated and incorporated into future planning processes.

We also must recognize that some diseases will be best treated by complementary or alternative medicine. Sound research data is supporting the facts that nontraditional medical procedures, long used successfully in other countries, are proving their value among Americans. Examples include the use of acupuncture for severe cases of tinnitus and migraine headaches. (26) One of the authors, Peter, who suffered from spondylolisthesis, sought out acupuncture as a last resort for severe pain when his traditional provider had gone skiing and was not available. He has been pain free ever since and that was 19 years ago. We don't know how it works, maybe the placebo effect, but it is what it is and he is a testament to it.

Events of trauma are increasing. Trauma is now the leading cause of death in people 65 years and younger, moving from the early teens just 20 years ago. (27) The reason is more diseases are being cured or controlled. Consequently, the aging population is, in many cases, healthier and therefore more prone to experiencing a traumatic event, perhaps even a life-ending one. This will require growth in trauma services, which today are often not profitable.

The number of infectious diseases is growing. (28) As international travel continues to grow, and mutations of bacteria and viruses are being identified, the number of cases of serious infectious diseases continues to rise. What this means for the organization with regard to staff and facilities will have to be considered as part of its future thinking.

Innovation must be encouraged. New approaches to treatments must be developed along with the advances and changing view of medicine in this country. For example, some forms of cancer are being removed from the American Cancer Society's list. (29) Acceptable blood pressure levels are being raised for people over 50. (30) Many health care professionals are now recognizing the overuse and misuse of prescription medications. (31)

## New Delivery Locations

In-patient volumes are continuing to decline in most markets. (32) This is predicted to continue, with the less acute patients being moved into ambulatory settings. This decline will be increasingly significant in locations where the population is not growing. We project that: hospital beds will be filled primarily with extremely ill, high-risk patients who need care from a relatively small number of service lines and, further, that hospitals will have to address enhanced infectious-disease-control processes, both for patients and visitors.

With this declining inpatient volume becoming the new norm, patients will be receiving more and more of their care and clinical services in non-acute settings and from non-traditional providers of care. (33-39) These include the following:

- Ambulatory Clinics. Hospitals will continue to increase their outpatient services, even converting some of their now-vacant inpatient floors to innovative outpatient services.
- New Entrants into the Market. Many geographical areas are seeing an increase in freestanding independent urgent-care centers, freestanding but hospital-connected emergency departments, and convenient clinics in retail stores, including pharmacies. The companies that own and operate such facilities have growth plans that, if successful, will continue to drive the market even more significantly away from hospital dominance.
- Telemedicine. The uses of telemedicine, especially by small and rural hospitals, is growing and expanding to numerous product lines beyond stroke, including dermatology and behavioral

services. The potential for this method of acquiring the correct diagnosis and treatment plans from offsite experts is unlimited.

- <u>Hospitals at Home</u>. More and more services can be provided in the home, and traditional home health agencies are now incorporating these into the menu of services they provide.
- <u>Palliative and Hospice Service</u>. Although increasingly used by all age groups, the elderly, when faced with a terminal disease, will quickly avail themselves of such services.
- <u>Wellness Centers</u>. The movement to population health will increase the focus on wellness and prevention of disease, driving the growth of these services in the future. They are often self-pay product lines, and hence, if managed appropriately, can be one of the few revenue growth opportunities available for the traditional hospital.
- <u>New National Treatment Centers</u>. Traditionally, treatment of burns has been handled best in a few well-established centers in the United States. That practice is being extended to other specialties. There is now a national center for cancer treatments, through dispersed regional locations, and similar plans are on the drawing board for cardiac and eye surgery centers of excellence.

**Financial Challenges**

It's a new day and age when it comes to paying for medical services. Following are a few of the financial challenges that systems need to consider:

- <u>Bundled Payments</u>. New forms of payment will be compensating physicians, hospitals and other providers. We will see one payment for an episode of patient care. Integrated models, such as that required for an accountable care organization, will be required to care for patients and to manage the distribution and allocation of payments. This will require a trust level in the future among all clinical care parties, which has rarely been achieved in the past.
- <u>Pay-for-Performance</u>. Perhaps the most jarring of changes will be pay-for-performance. If value versus volume is the mandate, then aligning incentives with more pay or rewards for better service will

be part of the future landscape. This is a pervasive change and will be a lasting marker of transformation in the history of healthcare.

- Declining Payment. Belts are tightening everywhere. There is downward pressure on the money available for care. Insurance companies and other related health care vendors are reluctant to see their profit margins decline. Consequently, traditional providers will have to deal with payments that are less each year, with little or no opportunities to grow their revenue lines.

- Enhanced and Total Transparency. If pay-for-performance is a reality, then being transparent with all aspects of care will be required, including clinical and service outcomes.

- Direct Contracting. Hospitals and physicians will attempt to contract directly with the insurers, encouraging them to support a narrow network of providers who have data to prove their care is better.

- The Costs of Information Technology (IT). Accurate data requires an effective information technology platform that can integrate care from all providers and be analyzed in real time. This requires large amounts of capital and will be a continuing high-cost area in the future.

- A Committed Workforce. The increasing financial pressures caused by declining volumes and revenues are resulting in staff pressure. While this is to be expected as part of any successful transformational journey, hospitals must simultaneously seek methods to improve physician and employee satisfaction and engagement. A committed and engaged workforce is a critical success factor for the future and can only be accomplished by establishing a strong culture and brand.

## Need for New Partners

Rather than being treated as their customers, hospitals will need to put in place tactics so physicians see a value in becoming partners with the hospital. They must embrace collaboration, and transformation strategies and tactics, for long-term success.

Given the new competition in the ambulatory markets, exploring ways to partner with these newcomers will be necessary.

## Evolving Physician Models

We've come a long way since the family doctor made house calls. Following are some of the more recent trends:

- Growth of Mixed Models. Although in the past, hospital systems either had employed models, such as Geisinger or Cleveland Clinic, or the independent practitioner model, most today have a mixed model of some employed physicians, traditional contracted physicians, hospitalists, and independent practitioners, which still make up the greatest number. This mixed model will not go away and will provide a challenge to hospital leaders as to how to bring this group together in a united physician voice.

- Physician Performance Goals. Given that physicians are the primary drivers of clinical outcomes, quality performance measures must be built into future employment contracts, and into the credentialing process for independent practitioners. Consequences for noncompliance must be communicated and enforced.

- New Hospitalists. Hospital-based physicians began with radiologists, pathologists, and, in some areas of the country, anesthesiologists and emergency room physicians. Now intensive-care providers, neonatologists, and general hospitalists are becoming quite common. In the future, obstetrical hospitalists as well as those trained to manage postoperative patients will become part this model of care. And just like the evolution of physician practices moving from solo practice models to larger and larger groups, hospitalists are now part of larger regional and even national hospitalist groups. Contractual negotiations with these groups requires increasing sophistication.

- Increase in Primary Care Providers. Integrated care must involve a strong component of primary care. With the shortage of primary care physicians, and with limited growth projected into the future, the use of physician extenders and nurse practitioners will markedly increase. State licensing boards, even in the face of some physician resistance, are increasingly expanding the allowable scope of practice to facilitate this future need.

The landscape for the future of health care is becoming clearer. There is much we know we need to do. Indeed, in this chapter, we have touched on some topics and themes that need to be addressed by every provider of health services. Of course, we also know that health care, given its immense size and impact on the entire economy of the United States is a huge political target, or should say: football. It is oddly shaped, bounces irregularly, it is difficult to hold onto, it captures our attention, but is frustrating and expensive. Any rational future must address structural delivery challenges-including insurance and other forms of coverage, quality initiatives and performance, but most of all, we advocate for a health care future that addresses the many social influences that contribute to unhealthy lives. Controversy is sure to be part of the future. Political rhetoric will abound. Changes to existing law will happen...again and again and again. If our experience is worth anything at all it is this: change happens, it is the nature of the future. So be a part of it in your organization, in your community, in the country...for the good of all.

# Chapter 5

# Implementing Successful Transformation Strategies

**"It's not only what we do, but also what we do not do, for which we are accountable," -- Moliere**

Based on personal experiences, presence in the field, and comparing high- and low-performing institutions, we know that successful organizations have three consistent transformational underpinnings, optimizing **collaboration** while minimizing competition, aligning **incentives** while eradicating a win/lose mentality, and demanding **accountability** for outcomes.

## COLLABORATION

For decades, a competitive model has driven the U.S. health care system. If hospital X promoted a new piece of equipment or new service, it was likely that hospital Y would quickly move to do the same. Physicians would threaten the administrators at hospital X that if they did not get what they wanted they would take their business, and hence hospital revenue, to hospital Y. Of course, this was aided and abetted by decades of legal opinions regarding the 'community standard'. This was a de facto form of pressure for all hospital providers to provide at or nearly so the same level of care and equipment as their competitor or risk being held accountable by a court for failure to adhere to the 'community standard of care'.

Competition is critical in environments where the customer pays the total cost of the product. It helps to ensure greater value through the rigor of a transparent marketplace. However, the American health care system is a unique service industry where customers pay little out-of-pocket, and are often limited to certain providers because of insurance policies or governmental regulations. The health care industry has been insulated from the economic principles driving the outcomes for other sectors.

For hospitals revenue-generating services are, increasingly, diminishing. Therefore, expenses must be reduced, while striving to maintain a high level of quality. While the industry experiences rapid declines in payments and acute-care volumes new entrants into the market steal valuable market share, so collaboration (or consolidation) rather than competition, becomes a growing key to transformational success.

This competitive model is one of the prime reasons for the many challenges in the industry. This model is no longer a workable strategy. It has toxic effects that tear down, rather than build up, an institution. Collaboration, working with others for the greater good, is like the tide that raises all boats. Collaboration addresses and corrects these fundamental flaws in the US *non-system* of healthcare:

- overcapacity of beds, and duplication of services in a geographical area
- overuse/misuse of diagnostic and treatment modalities
- treating physicians as customers
- friction between physicians and hospitals
- overlooking patient and community priorities
- the belief that to survive, someone must fail
- no recognition that other community health and wellness assets have value

## Acting Like a System

A collaborative environment must first and foremost be enhanced internally in any organization if it is to be successful today. The challenges are so complex that the solutions must evolve from the collective brainpower of the team members. Working in silos and reporting upward in strong vertical lines has been the tradition in the health care industry. But, one-way, top-down communication is debilitating. Critical functions must be carried out horizontally by multidisciplinary teams that are comfortable working in a matrix reporting structure. This change requires health care services organizations to function as an integrated system internally. In the past, in the competitive model, system-ness might have meant standardized letterhead, signage and group purchasing. Today, full collaboration across all parts of the system, both clinically and administratively, must be implemented. We discuss this more fully in Chapter Eleven.

## A Cohesive Leadership Team

Collaborative decision making, which is critical in designing and implementing the organization's future road map, requires a cohesive leadership team which will be further discussed in another chapter.

## Uniform Understanding of Clinical Integration

Regardless whether the Affordable Care Act stands or falls, partially or entirely, organizations today must assume accountability for the care that they are providing. In reality, this was the intent of the managed-care programs beginning with the very first HMO legislation in the 1970's. The potential and innovative notions of managing care became a managed payment mechanism based on risk, rather than an integrated approach to supporting and promoting the health status of a defined population.

Success in clinical integration requires the following:

- multi-disciplinary teams driving coordination of care across the entire continuum
- financial penalties and rewards determined by outcome metrics

- agreement that the only acceptable care is that which is high quality, safe, affordable, and accessible
- developing a workable bundled payment process with all delivery partners
- evidence-based medical protocols to reduce variations in outcomes
- best practices creating efficiencies in administrative procedures being developed and transported throughout the organization

## Building and Respecting Referral Networks

A strong relationship with all primary-care physicians and midlevel providers, whose numbers will increase as they are hired to staff more and more services, should be high on the CEO's priority list.

Forging strong relationships with specialists is also important because it is likely their referrals will increase. Because of their rising insurance rates, and threats of medical malpractice lawsuits, specialists will be less likely to do borderline cases. Hence, they will refer their more complicated patients to hospitalists.

Pinched by higher-deductible insurance plans, people will choose to conduct online research and self-refer to the hospital and physicians that they think will provide the best value services. These reshaping and evolving referral patterns should drive a transformational marketing and communication plan that will result in a seamless referral process, replacing the often-bumpy road known in too many facilities.

## Determining Your New Partners

Transitioning from a competitive to a collaborative model requires exploring all potential partnerships that could be developed, even with old competitors. Together, decisions can be made collectively as to where the most comprehensive array of services would best be provided. Their combined efforts should also increase affordability and accessibility, both enhancing the integrated brand and leading to growth and sustainability.

The menus of potential partnership considerations should, at minimum, include: affiliation of programs, shared services, integration of services, a full legal merger/consolidation and acquisition of assets.

Regardless of the degree of the partnership, it requires agreement and collaborative behaviors among all parties, which is dependent on picking the right partner at the onset of the discussions. Desired characteristics are compatible values and strong brand.

**Partnering with Medical Staff**

Physicians are the primary driver of the quality and safety of clinical outcomes. Of course, they must work in concert with nurses and other members of the health care team. Additionally, physicians control the accessibility of appropriate care by the degree they limit their office hours, the number of patients they are willing to see per session, and the insurance types they will accept. Because of this, hospitals and health systems must transform the physician relationship from customer to partner. Together health care organizations and physicians can create and implement solutions to ongoing and future challenges.

Physicians are also critical drivers of the cost of the various health care products and treatment modalities. Therefore, they must develop a significant ownership and accountability for both aspects of the value equation—quality over cost.

Any effort to transform the nature, scope or character of any health care institution must secure the collaboration of the physicians associated with that institution. Not doing so ensures a wasted effort no matter how noble.

**Enhancing Staff Engagement**

Having satisfied physicians, and employees, is not adequate today for a successful transformation. Rather, they must be engaged in their work, which means all staff have a heightened emotional connection to their organization and leaders, which drives them to excellent work and outcomes.

Tips to enhance engagement include the following:

- frequently reminding staff of the importance of their work
- being clear, both verbally and in writing, about work expectations and metrics of success
- offering pathways for professional development and advancement
- believing in the ethics, mission, vision, and values of the organization and living them out daily
- being credible (walking the talk)
- providing regular effective, comprehensive, and transparent communications
- recognizing and rewarding personnel

Engaged physicians and employees are collaborative, aligned and accountable. They support and drive the strategies of transformational success.

## Aligned Incentives

If the competitive model has fueled most of the major challenges in the health care industry today, misaligned incentives between the hospital or health system and their physicians and staff is the second major culprit. If designing and implementing the road map to success requires the brainpower of many, then aligning the incentives among all stakeholders, creating a win/win environment, is indeed a critical strategy to drive transformational success.

In the past, many events occurred that polarized the players needed to work together in a true partnership. These win/lose activities must be named and eliminated.

Implementation of the Diagnostic-Related Group (DRG) payment system, as an unintentional consequence, incentivized hospitals to discharge patients quickly. This put them in an oppositional posture to attending physicians because the physician had no incentive for early discharge. In fact, early-on in the DRG payment system, the physician still had financial incentives to keep the patient in the hospital. This, coupled with the desire of the doctor to ensure that all the best possible care was provided to the patient, meant that the doctors and hospitals were at odds regarding when it was best to discharge a patient. Over time, as the length of hospital stay decreased for patients based on the DRG payment system it also contributed to reducing concurrent daily charges for physicians. Doctors were not happy campers.

Government payment policies, driven by a need to balance the budget, often shifted around hospital and physician payments thus creating a conflicting relationship between physicians and hospitals. To restore income and regain some control of their patients, some doctors acquired what were once only hospital technologies, such as CTs and MRIs. These were placed in medical offices or physician-owned outpatient centers that, in turn, reduced the hospital's revenue stream. The increasing tenuous relationships among all those involved in-patient care activities led to rigidity and lines drawn in the sand.

The more formalized relationship between hospitals and providers resulted in a lack of willingness to share data that could have helped identify best practices and, indeed, eliminated other questionable practices that should have been changed in the name of quality care. There has been little to no interconnectivity of information technologies so clinical data could be shared easily, and duplications of some tests and information which could be eliminated. Though recent efforts to improve this have been implemented and incentivized through payment policies, there is still a long, long way to go.

Hospital leadership had, and still has, a tendency to solicit, reward, and entice physicians who had the best potential for enhancing the growth and/ or success of the hospital. This furthered the competitive model of behavior between physicians and the hospital and likewise, between physicians themselves.

To overcome these long-established and well-embedded conditions that have driven polarization, transformational leaders must focus on the following key initiatives to develop alignment among all the stakeholders in the health care industry.

## Transparency

Total transparency is mandatory. It is now a public expectation and without it, an institution of any sort is suspect. Full candor, including metrics of success and clinical outcomes, builds trust. It is only by being honest about where an organization is that a leader can align incentives with the appropriate people who have the skill and will to guide the organization on the road to success. Transparency of results, down to the individual performance level, must be made visible to the internal stakeholders as well as to the external community. One of the authors, Jay, wrote in an internet article regarding his experience with metrics that measurement as a tool to ensure desired progress and success could also lead to manipulation of the numbers. Leaders must never lose their moral compass where honesty is always true north. People follow dishonest leaders only if they have to, never because they want to. Transparency requires integrity.

## Effective Information Technology

The availability of and sharing of real-time, accurate data is critical for proper alignment. Effective and reliable information technology, processing both clinical and administrative data, is essential for success. Effective information technology may be expensive, and the return on the investment is not always immediately apparent. The solutions to today's health care challenges can only be developed by informed leaders who drive the implementation of successful solutions based on knowledge and data from a strong IT platform.

## Setting Physician Expectations

Inasmuch as the physician is most often the leader in the clinical setting, the physician staff, whether employed or independent, must be aligned with the organization's goals. One of the greatest barriers to transformational strategies occurs when physicians are held to a different (usually lower) level of accountability. Performance expectations must be built into the contracts of employed and hospital-based physicians, as well as into the re-credentialing process for independent practitioners. These expectations, with success metrics, must address productivity, clinical and safety outcomes, service delivery and patient satisfaction, team leadership and behaviors and participation in cost-saving initiatives.

## Physicians as Partners

As with all employees and staff, the physicians must have aligned incentives if they are to become true partners. Physicians are committed to doing what is best, in collaboration with the health system, for the community they jointly serve. Alignment of effort is a duty for all.

One important initiative for alignment is the development of a physician compact. Written by a task force populated by physicians and administrative leaders, this document itemizes what the organization expects of its physicians, and what the physicians should expect from the organization. By posting and reviewing this document periodically to determine the degree of compliance, both parties continue their mutual commitment, built on a trustful relationship. We implemented a physician compact at CHRISTUS hospitals. Was it easy? No. Was it important? Yes. One of the greatest benefits came from the dialogue and engagement between health system leaders and practicing physicians. The resulting compacts, promises really, expressed the time tested and relational basis of the institution and physician commitments. These documents, while not a legal contract by any means, did form a moral basis for desired behaviors and expectations.

## Recognition of High Performance

High performers constantly strive to exceed expectations. If they are treated no differently than those employees who are content with mediocre outcomes even well motivated people will eventually wonder if they are beating their heads against the wall. High performers have an innate sense of duty and commitment that gives them a high degree of intrinsic motivation. But over time, if not recognized, even this can wear thin and they will decide it is not worth it and they will seek other opportunities. To prevent this from happening, recognition programs, or incentive pay-for-performance, must be made available to all who on a regular basis exceed their goals. Conversely, everyone needs to understand what the consequences will be if the expectations are not met or, even worse, ignored. Incentives work best when they are carrots. Mediocre employees rarely are motivated by anything, not the carrot nor the stick. They must be dealt with appropriately or risk losing the best talent to a competitor.

## Accountability

Leaders, by their actions, must behave according to their defined company values. Solid leaders should maintain a daily focus on the mission and vision, communicating them as often as possible, to serve as the guide to developing the transitional road map to the future. Walking the talk drives, more than anything else, leadership credibility.

## Clarity of Goals and Expectations

Performance expectations and goals must be developed and implemented at every level: the board, CEO, leadership team, all departments, service line, and employees.

The degree of success, to reach these goals, must be monitored on a regular basis. Corrective action plans must be developed for those that are off target. Discussion about goals must be the center point of the periodic review process for all employees, regardless of role. These sessions should include a conversation about the competencies that are required to meet these goals and those of the future. For any competencies that are deemed less than adequate, a performance improvement plan should be developed, and agreed upon, to close the performance gap.

Most people are hired because whoever is doing the recruitment believes the individual can perform the roles and responsibilities outlined in the job description. Unfortunately, after the hire, monitoring and measuring expected outcomes and metrics of success are often lacking.

A well-written job description is clear. It defines expectations unambiguously. Rarely does the job description detail how an employee is to fulfill the role, or more importantly, define the measurements for success. While agreeing to roles and responsibilities is important, an employee will, most likely, perform only satisfactory work if expectations are not clear or challenging.

Within the modern health care environment, satisfactory outcomes are not adequate for achieving sustainability and transformational success. Meeting and surpassing goals are no longer a luxury but a necessity. Staff who adhere to and reflect a culture of accountability most readily achieve goals.

High performing employees are accountable employees. They are never pleased with satisfactory outcomes. These individuals strive continuously to do the very best they can do. As a consequence, they do meaningful work and often are the key drivers of transformational processes. They embrace and are energized to reach stretch goals that accelerate the organization's journey to excellence. They are constantly open to learning new and better ways to achieve the highest levels of operational performance. This optimal level of performance comes from reducing variability in both clinical and administrative processes and outcomes. In organizations that are only marginally successful, variability in quality, safety, and transparency is most often identified as a key concern.

Well-defined goals, with metrics of success, are the crux of accountability. They must be present at all levels of the organization for future success. These must emanate from the top of the organization with the board, CEO and the senior leadership team all in agreement. Accountability drives improvement in quality and safety, service delivery, and financial outcomes.

Chapter 6

# Implementing a Strong Culture and Brand

**"Branding demands commitment; commitment to continual re-invention; striking chords with people to stir their emotions; and commitment to imagination." – Sir Richard Branson**

## Culture Trumps Strategy

Based upon articles and interviews with C-suite teams, a significant number of hospitals and health systems are either in, or believe they are headed to, a performance crisis. Clearly, if successful turnarounds in these organizations are going to occur, everyone working there must coalesce around a common vision, utilizing their best efforts to reach agreed-upon improvement metrics, particularly around quality, service and costs. Such outcomes ultimately require a common culture among all stakeholders, including board members, the CEO, leadership and management teams, physicians, and, perhaps even most important, all the employees in the organization.

Although the importance of creating such an environment may not be fully understood and embraced, culture always trumps strategy. In essence, these critical words, perhaps a nicety in the past, are now an essential component of a thriving organization. If the desired culture of an organization is not embraced and espoused by its employees, the best strategies for sustainable success, even if well implemented, may fail. The culture is the soul of the company and its people and the right people drive the right outcomes.

For many decades, the measure of greatness for any hospital or health system was often equated to the amount of its real estate and it relative size. The size and number of its bed towers, the number of services offered, the amount of revenue generated, the size of the workforce, and being the first in the community to acquire the newest technologies were markers of importance. The phrase: "the bigger the better" implied that their people—their quality, brainpower, and competencies—were not the company's major asset, size was.

All of this does not mean that there was not an underlying culture in the organization. What it does mean is that, for leadership, the development and enhancement of a strong and vibrant culture and brand were not a high priority on the to-do list. In fact, the culture of the organization was often taken for granted. Leaders typically say they have a great culture. But, when asked to define its components and the strategies used to achieve it, the responses are shallow and lack substance. The answers often include the fact that most of the physicians are happy, turnover of the staff is acceptable, and a good operating margin is being achieved.

After some investigation, we often find that true physician involvement, both in generating input and participating in decision-making, is limited. Many physicians see themselves as customers of the hospital whose needs and wants, because they are the revenue generators, have to be satisfied. With a bit of arrogance, some may even state that they are the culture of the organization. Sadly, this perception may have been abetted by an organizational and its leadership deference to, rather than a partnership with, physicians. We have seen this first hand. It is extremely difficult to change a culture when a key partner, like a doctor, has created an aura of invincibility, lives with an attitude of entitlement and this aberrant behavior has been tolerated by management. Such a toxic combination can undermine an organizational culture and destroy employee morale. But if addressed quickly and decisively, with respect for all, employees notice. Other doctors notice. The board notices. Peter had to deal with this shortly after assuming leadership in one of our hospitals. A physician who had practiced at this institution almost his entire career had a well earned reputation for consistently being verbally abusive to the nursing staff, to other hospital based physicians and, also, on occasion he would press the envelope of the limit of his clinical competency. He had been reviewed many times by the medical staff, but little action had been taken. This was no doubt complicated by the fact that he was ranked as one of the top three admitters to the hospital. Finally, after many consultations with a new chief medical officer and with the careful review and documentation of information from patient records and from other sources, this doctor received his due process from the medical staff review committee and the hospital but, eventually, he was removed from the medical staff. Of course, he appealed to the Board of Directors for and received a thorough review of the circumstances surrounding his dismissal. The Board upheld the decision of the medical staff. He asked for yet another review directly with Peter and requested that several of his physician friends be allowed to accompany him to this meeting. To make a long story short, near the end of this meeting, at which all of the related matters regarding his dismissal were again reviewed, this doctor emptied his pockets of change and keys and assorted objects and began throwing them at Peter. His physician friends (who also admitted to the hospital) were shocked. The doctor had lost all of his remaining support. What was the result of all of this? The hospital lost a substantial amount of revenue due to the loss of this doctors admissions, but the nursing staff and other professional staff saw a new standard, a new culture, that was being established; other physicians also noticed. Clinical professionalism and accountability was not only talk, it was undergirded with action. Cultural standards can be established, written, discussed, and presented ad nauseam, but they are earned every day.

Can an organization have measurable success without a vibrant and strong culture? Often leaders point to financial success as the measure of ultimate success. A good margin can hide problems but these problems will eventually, just like a rust spot under the paint on a car, find their way to the surface as a much larger issue. Some markers for issues which can be ignored at managements peril include a sudden rise in staff turnover, difficulty hiring the right staff, young physicians deciding that they will seek privileges elsewhere, and others. Markers like these can be ignored and glossed over in the short term by defensive management behaviors, but they cannot be ignored for long.

## What Does Cultural Transformation Look Like?

In the April 2009 edition of Health Leaders magazine, Carrie Vaugh's article "The Bumpy Road to Change," (40) refers to cultural change as that "unambiguous phrase seemingly at the heart of every hospital turnaround effort, quality improvement program, or employment satisfaction initiative." Vaugh points out that because cultural transformation is so difficult, many of these efforts are failing. Her observations substantiate and support the belief of many that an organization's culture is its trump card. Most successful leaders and board chairs today would quickly agree that the best strategies will not be implemented if the culture of the company is not fully understood and embraced by all the staff. They know the culture is what makes the strategies work, what makes the organization's heart tick. It is a major requirement of leadership to ensure that a good sustaining culture is established and maintained.

Knowing this is not enough. Implementation is critical in this complex and challenging period in health care. The culture of the organization must be the platform upon which a clear and rational strategic plan can rest. Each strategy must have implementable tactics, each with well-defined outcome goals, performance metrics, responsible individuals or teams for achievement, and defined timelines for expected completion. This means the culture demands a high level of accountability for all people in whatever role they are playing. As stated earlier, most companies do a relatively good job of creating job descriptions, clearly defining employees' roles and responsibilities. However, clear communication of the performance expectations and accountability metrics is often lacking. A thriving culture has, as one of its bedrocks, a strong commitment to a high level of accountability within its ranks.

Because the company's culture is so critical for a successful transformation, it must not be known only to its internal staff but also must be recognizable by its existing and potential customers. To an external audience, culture becomes the company's brand. Both the culture and the brand are made up of those ingredients and characteristics that, if they went away, would make the company's products and services unrecognizable and, more importantly, no longer desirable. Brands are weakened by the degree of variability in their products. Variability, the lack of continual and predictable clinical and service efficacy, is a significant issue present in the health care delivered today. If the brand is not stronger than that of a competitor, why would an organization expect its services to be desired and its sustainability to be secured?

Cultural transformation, to be successful, requires that the mission, vision and values of the organization be robust, relevant, lived out and supported daily by every member of the staff and board. These are, as previously stated, the who, where and how of the company's culture. They are the foundational building blocks and the brand of the company, and they drive the performance of its people, leading to growth, innovation and long-term sustainability.

Competent leadership is also critical for true cultural transformation to occur. Transformation of any organization starts at the top. Leaders must instill, cultivate, nurture, and fortify their organization's culture. They must fully understand each component of the culture and the brand, and clearly communicate that the support of such is nonnegotiable. The leader must recognize that little can be accomplished, alone. They must have not only a strong team committed to the culture and brand but team members who, in turn, demand the same level of commitment from the members of their teams. This approach must filter through the entire organization, so each and every board member, leader, director, manager, and employee clearly understands his or her role in building and maintaining the culture and brand that are critical to the company's success.

## Barriers to a Strong Culture and Brand

If a strong culture and brand are critical success factors for every health care organization in these challenging times, why is establishing and maintaining a vibrant culture not on many CEOs' list of priorities?

Some leaders believe cultural development in their organization will occur automatically, if everything else is done correctly. Unfortunately, the opposite may be true. Success creates confidence. An organization, like an individual, can become overconfident. Complacency can creep in and, when it does, mediocre performance can be the consequence. Mediocrity is a destructive force. It undermines character and poisons the soul of an organization. It is dangerous to the construction of a culture of excellence. Some leaders view culture as having a low priority in comparison to harder strategies, like achieving financial success. Hence, it gets little attention or leadership emphasis. Such leaders will never fully realize the ultimate potential of their organization.

The health care environment is complex and challenging. Focusing on the business needs, improving clinical outcomes and safety, and dealing with other daily crises often leave little time for the leader to do cultural reflection and uninterrupted thinking. This lack of focus is always dangerous, but is especially so when leaders and boards are contemplating a merger or acquisition. When bringing together two organizations, the cultural fit should be of the highest priority. An honest cultural assessment of both organizations can often fall to the wayside when the details of a transaction overwhelm the best intentions. The majority of attention is often spent figuring out how being part of a bigger entity will make each partner better. In the end, it is the lack of cultural compatibility that becomes the reason a large number of potentially great business mergers end up failing.

Analysis of failed mergers have proven over and over again that the prior reputations of each player can be weakened if each potential partner does not fully commit to supporting and agreeing on those factors that will determine the new company's brand identity. (41) This is always more challenging than originally thought, especially when each party has well-ingrained traditions, some for 50 to 100 years. The difficulty in bringing the organizations together and developing a common culture and brand can be compared to the challenges faced if a couple adopted an 18-year-old and attempted to meld him or her seamlessly into their well-established family. The 18-year-old, without a strong commitment from all family members to patiently teach the family's values and role model the family's culture, may never assimilate as the other children who were raised from infancy.

Components of the brand must be explored, discussed and agreed upon. Before collaborative agreements are signed for shared services, partnership with insurance companies, or full legal mergers or consolidations with other health care institutions all the salient aspects of an organization's culture and brand must be candidly revealed and discussed. The goal of completing a 'deal' must not override the foundational aspects of the organizations making the deal.

It is important to note that internal competition can result when agreement is not reached to support each of these components of the brand. Pressure to outperform others will often drive a person to lose their moral compass and begin participating in actions that are lacking integrity and honesty. That is why a strong level of organizational ethics must be incorporated into the culture and brand of a successful organization. The comfort that this will occur also is embedded in another critical component of the culture, creating a climate of non-retaliation.

All members of the work-family must be comfortable in telling each other and the leaders what they need to hear about the realities they are experiencing. Candor and professional pushback is not only important it is necessary. Almost every business sector now recognizes the value of candid, yet respectful, dialogue among all levels of an organization as a critical success factor. Sugarcoating information and telling the leaders only what they want to hear is dangerous for the organization's health. Successful leaders will accept reality. Dr. Tom was famous in several of the organizations he served because he would invite professional pushback by saying: "you can argue with me, challenge me and call me idiotic, but when I start to cry you have to back-off". Humor is always good to break down barriers. Most leaders find meaning in difficult situations; they make continuous plans for a better future, and move quickly to solve problems; they develop innovative strategies and develop and support processes that result in rapid implementation.

## Staying Focused on Culture and Brand

It is easy to understand why health care leaders, faced with multiple large-scale challenges, including: pay-for-performance, value-based purchasing, inpatient volume declines, coordinated care, integration of physicians, and population-health management, find it easy to ignore their organization's culture. Yet, because it is well known that culture drives strategies, and strategies and their tactics drive outcome; ignoring the basic need for a strong organizational cultural is foolhardy.

The focus on creating and maintaining a strong culture and brand must be intentional, and given a high priority. Processes and behaviors to accomplish this must be put in place.

At our last organization, we were challenged by two different layers of the same cake. We had formed a very large system through the consolidation of two other long-established smaller systems. This was not an acquisition; one group was not being melded and subsumed into another. A new culture had to be established which was "owned by all". At the same time, the two smaller systems that we were consolidating on a much larger scale were made up of several smaller regionally based and geographically identified sub-systems and/or separate hospitals. These regional systems had cultural and branding pressures of their own most often caused by market dynamics and competitive issues locally. We had to figure out a way to establish not only a new cultural identity while being faithful to the historical and faith traditions of the founding sponsors, but we had to shore up the identities of the established operators in their local markets.

Talk is easy, too easy. Culture is a lived value and so must be brought to life everyday through action. Doing so is not easy, but is critical. As the CEO of this new system, Dr. Tom was visible in the field and visiting with team members. The formative process begins with leadership. The CEO, leadership team members and physician leaders must, above all, be authentic. They must role model the values of the organization daily, and do what they say they are going to do. We discovered by making rounds frequently (though in a large multi-state organization, making "rounds" required almost daily travel to a distant location) that presence, while important, was not enough. We needed to shape the culture and establish the brand through a consistent and well thought out educational program that emphasized our identity, mission, and values. Our system-wide educational program for cultural identity ensured consistency across the entire organization and throughout its many facets: local leadership, medical staff, local governing boards, community members and became the basis for a unified image as well as recognition. Education is more than training, it includes the concept of dialogue, of listening and exchanging ideas. Our commitment to the entire health system was to lead, but also to listen, to receive input from those who served people everyday. It is interesting to note that the word listen is made up of the same letters as the word silent. Leaders need not be always speaking, they need to be quiet and listen. We did this. We learned a lot from those who were on the line every day. In this way, we also demonstrated the respect for others that was one of our espoused values. Leaders set the tone and are responsible for establishing the culture needed for organizational success. One of our cultural cornerstones was that each employee, who we later termed an associate, was to know that they were heard, valued and respected in their own right. They were valued for their professionalism and skill, and we measured and scored their competencies as a gauge for them to understand their own contributions to the overall success of the organization; but they were also valued in their own right as fellow servants in our health ministry. We reminded them frequently of the intersection of their professionalism and their own humanity when we said, to them as well as ourselves, that we were blessed each day to care for the greatest gift anyone could receive… the gift of another person's life in our hands and in our care. Culture is like most other aspects of organizational life and it requires constant assessment and support. We believe that institutional risk management programs should include the evaluation of the strength of its culture and brand. We also programmed culture attributes and expectations as a key part of our internal as well as external communications. And, truth be known, we did a lot of communication inside and outside of the organization.

When establishing the CHRISTUS brand, we knew this would, just like establishing a culture, need to be more than talk. Most people think of a brand as the external expression of the organization; some would say-culture is the inside game and brand is the outside game. A brand is more than a logo; it is more than tag lines in a marketing program; it is more than uniforms and color schemes- your brand is what people think of you. One of the authors, Peter, spent seven years working on a large cattle ranch. Every spring calves were branded. This brand was meant to dignify ownership of the animal; and also, was the sign to other ranchers that this cow or bull or calf belonged on that specific ranch. But to the rancher, the brand was more than a mark and more than a claim, it was also a reputation for, as other cattlemen saw and assessed that animal, they also judged the rancher who owned it. This is the power of a brand. Your reputation, and therefore your credibility and success, depend upon it. A story regarding our brand was sent to us in a letter from a former patient. This man had relatives traveling within our hospital geography and told them that if they needed a hospital or healthcare services to look for the CHRISTUS logo and name. He was sure that the excellent care he had received would be consistently available wherever one of our facilities was located. This is the power of a brand. We worked hard to develop it, to get our employees to understand the components of our brand and to maintain it. A standard among those in the marketing business is that if a person has a positive experience with a business they will tell another, sometimes even two persons. But if they have a negative experience, they will tell nine people. Your brand and your reputation is in the hearts of your customers.

When it comes to establishing a brand, we are strong advocates for augmenting your own instincts, desires, traditions and values with the technical expertise of outside experts. Companies like Scorpion, which specializes in internet marketing and brand identity and The Write Counsel, which specializes in the more traditional print and media fields are excellent examples of experts which can assist healthcare organizations improve their brand. The most recent U.S. presidential election is proof positive of the power of brand and the use of social media.

## A Checklist for Culture and Brand

- The CEO must agree that cultural formation begins with them. But, unlike most CEO's temperament, they must be patient because cultural change is a long time commitment.
- The CEO, leadership team members and physician leaders must, above all, be authentic. They must role model the values of the organization on a daily basis, and do what they say they are going to do.
- An ongoing educational program must be developed and implemented for both employees and new hires, articulating the importance of the culture and their role in support and strengthening it.
- Assure that the values are fully understood and lived out on a daily basis by building a review of such into everyone's annual performance evaluation. This type of review should also be included in the re-credentialing process for all physicians, whether independent, contracted, or employed.
- People should know they are valued in the organization, and the success of the organization depends on their performance. Enlist their input. Listen to their feedback. Involve them in decision-making, where possible. These processes develop ownership, and it is a well-known fact that owners take their roles much more seriously than employees.
- Develop constant communication plans regarding the organization's mission and values. It is important to note that most directors of communications believe that when you think you have communicated something enough, you should communicate it one more time.
- Utilize mission, vision and value statements as guidelines when making important decisions to assure these foundational building blocks will not be weakened.

- Insist on transparency in everything, especially in reporting on outcome data in clinical and administrative areas.
- Demand a high level of accountability to both individuals and teams, comparing on a regular basis their performance results to the predetermined success metrics.
- Clearly delineate the components of the organization's brand, which must be maintained consistently to keep it recognizable.
- Consider implementing a system-wide organizational ethics program to minimize the potential of the workforce losing their moral compass.
- Design a system-wide enterprise risk program to encourage the staff to not only identify the potential risks with new endeavors but also develop action plans to mitigate the risks to whatever degree possible. This will help preclude the barriers to transformational change.
- Remember that meaningful transformational strategies may take time, and the change process may have to be evolutionary versus revolutionary. However, in today's environment, speed must be guided by the urgency of the amount of fire on the burning platform.
- Remind staff to come in each day and remember that patients turn over to them their most precious gifts -- their lives. This is an awesome responsibility that underscores that excellence is not a luxury but a necessity.

## Monitoring the Culture and the Brand

Although the culture of the organization may be hard to define, there are strategies and processes that can be implemented to assure that the essential components of the culture and brand are in place. Implementation is the key to success. This being the case, how do we know that the culture and brand is alive and well, visible to both the internal and external stakeholders? The answer ... by putting in place processes to monitor the degree of implementation of the culture and brand-building strategies.

One of the very first things we did when we combined two health systems into one was to ensure that our business processes and especially the decision matrix we used to make significant business or clinical decisions included two questions: First, how will this considered action or partner or purchase [or whatever] maintain or enhance our mission? Second, will this enhance our values and strengthen the likelihood of achieving our vision? Clearly, living into the authenticity of our stated mission/vision/values required specific behaviors and chief among these was the "time out"; a time for team and personal reflection. We used a specific tool, a guideline, which ensured that we had obtained enough information and then used enough time to properly assess our decision-making quality and the ethical frame upon which it was based.

Another behavior we held ourselves to was, what we have mentioned as a critical aspect of high performing employees, accountability. Culture and brand are just like any other aspect of your services. Operational and financial performance are expected to be measured…sometimes daily. As we ensure accountability across the board for all aspects of the business, this very act restates, reinvigorates and strengthens the culture and brand. By acting professionally and competently in regard to stated goals, tactics, behavioral expectations, we, in turn, by proxy measure processes that ensure the integrity of the culture and brand. We also do this more formally. In our organization, we used specific tools developed to assess organizational culture. These are most often in the form of employee surveys, but other research techniques, validated and tested, have been used and we found them useful. The gauge for brand is customer surveys, perception/comparison studies, name recognition assessments, and many other tools. These are used throughout business in every segment. Building and maintaining a strong culture and brand requires constant attention. We thought about it every day because we knew if we did not all we were trying to do would disappear quickly

A strong culture and brand are so critical to transformational success that they should be the topics of conversations in many forums, both formal and informal, on a regular basis. Building and maintaining a strong culture and brand requires constant attention. If not top of mind, it may fade quickly.

By now it should be clear that the culture of the organization is how that day was lived out, how the day's challenges were addressed, how the end points were achieved, how the war was fought. A thriving culture and brand does not mean that operational outcomes are not important. It is known that even with a poor culture, the organization can still win the war, but in the end, many of the people will be "killed" in the process. If any of the good people are lost, celebrating the victories will become hollow. Most importantly, there will be many fewer good people willing to fight the next battle. This will be a sign that the culture is dying and that achieving excellence is in doubt.

## Chapter 7

# Excellence in Governance

**"To Change Something, Build a New Model That Makes the Old Model Obsolete," -- Buckminster Fuller**

**Building a Solid, Successful Board**

As health care organizations face the many transformational strategies that must be implemented as part of their road map to success, hospital and health system boards must evolve to provide excellence in governance. Many boards are still doing work that could be classified as titular, approving almost unanimously the recommendations of the CEO, with little review of supporting data. The role of a board member is not to rubber-stamp management's recommendations. This behavior must be transformed so the governance process is led by trustees who can expand their thinking well beyond the set of traditional policies and, often superficial, oversight functions.

The board is a critical player in the transformational journey to oversee the traditional outcome-oriented operations; but they also must help drive strategies that will ensure long-term success. Governance is critical for visionary and generative thinking. These responsibilities will keep the organization open to what the next transformation may need to be.

Fortunately, excellence in governance, which is lacking in many organizations, can be learned, incorporating principles and best practices that drive positive outcomes and forward momentum. Excellent governance, like competent leaders and cohesive and effective leadership teams, does not occur by accident. It must be an intentional board goal-clearly established, written and measured, just like the things the board expects of management, it must expect of itself in order be supportive and assure itself that the transformational strategies of the organization are implemented as necessary. This learning process takes time and must be planned, monitored, reviewed, and updated as necessary.

Good governance creates policy and strategic direction that support leadership and management in being successful at reaching their transformational operational and strategic directions. Poor governance has been shown to be a key element in the disabling of attempts to move an organization forward. As difficult as it may seem to be, poor governance practices must be identified, transparently surfaced for all to see and replaced with proven, effective governance practices.

## Creating Excellence in Governance

The first step in creating excellence in the governance is being aware of the barriers that prevent it from being supportive for the organization. With this knowledge, the board, the CEO and the leadership team, working as partners, can adopt and implement the best governance practices. Governance processes in health care have been in place for decades, as such they may be the type of practices, habits and comfortably hazy –even dysfunctional- behaviors that are not appropriate for today's dynamic and turbulent times. Let's examine common barriers that are standing in the way of creating governance excellence.

Traditionally, two major criteria for the selection of board members has been the importance of their professional job title or place in the community and their ability to make recurring financial donations. In addition, in public hospitals, where board members are often appointed by other governmental agencies, the trustees' appointments are often politically motivated. In the public domain where trustees are elected by community vote, popularity, not competence, often determines who will be the next person on the board directors. Other drivers of board appointments include longstanding friendships, social networks and business relationships. These same bonding factors can become obstacles in the boardroom. They foster decision-making driven by relationships rather than through careful consideration and objective analysis of data and measurable outcomes.

Relationships also lead much of the board work to be done, inappropriately, outside the boardroom, based on one-to-one exchanges between or among other trustees. In public boards these conversations are often illegal, but they occur anyway. Closed conversations provide the unhealthy opportunity for the CEO, or other board members, to get their personal agendas accomplished without taking into consideration what is best for the organization. Consequently, when all convene for the board meeting, some decisions may have been predetermined, and positions are not easily changed based on any honest discussion and objective data.

It would be wrong to suggest that the majority of board members, who are charged with governing our hospital delivery systems, are not well intentioned and wanting to make the right decisions and drive the right strategies. However, because they are often chosen without regard to whether or not they have the competencies to be excellent board members, they participate in what are mediocre governance processes at best. In addition, they frequently do not receive adequate information to serve as a basis for knowledge-driven decision making, or if they do, they do not understand what they have read. Nor, do they ask the right questions in meetings where there is little encouragement for robust discussions or disagreements. Trust in management is critical, but in some instances, it can be based on blind faith created by social relationships that spill over into the boardroom.

Although one of the major functions of a board is to provide oversight to the organization and the CEO, some board members may insert themselves inappropriately into day-to-day management. Oversight of management is not management—it is governance being aware, taking a look-that is: being watchful, seeking answers as needed, exercising responsibility!! Interacting with employees in the workplace, asking them what is really going on, assuring the employees they can make things better and even, in some instances, giving the employees direction is inappropriate. This has gone on without management's knowledge or counsel in many organizations. These board members are attempting to step in to resolve issues that are the responsibility of the CEO and the leadership team. Such action by a board member is counterproductive and must be censured.

Board members, well meaning though they may be, can also exceed appropriate boundaries in areas that are neither management nor governance exclusively. An example of this is when a board member may be a part of a strategic initiative or negotiation. Several years ago, we were involved in negotiating a very delicately balanced and sensitive, but potentially significant merger, between one of our entities and another health system in a local market. We made the decision that, for the purpose of greater unity with and respect for the local institution, the team involved in negotiations would include the local CEO and the local board chair. We were experienced and seasoned at the many different layers of dialogue, discourse and data required by merger negotiations; indeed, these layers can be complex and frustrating and they often take a long time to process and understand. In this context, the local board chair's frustration grew with the pace of the dialogue. The nature of a team, whether it be in business, medicine, sports or whatever, is that team unity most often results in the best outcome; the only exception to this that we have seen is in the actions of a medal of honor winner or a superstar athlete. In this case the board chair decided to act on his own and, unaware to other members of the negotiating team, contacted the board chair of the other entity. Their dialogue resulted in information shared that was compromising to our position and specific indications were made (though not promises) that our posture on certain issues could be amended. When we discovered the nature of these conversations and the reframed perceptions of the other party, we realized that the board chair had essentially scuttled the possibility of this transaction by violating our trust and instilling confusion in the other party. The intent was well meaning, the effort was sincere, but- in this case- the actions were outside the realm of the governance role. Unilateral behavior, no matter how noble or heroically minded, is fraught with risk. The upshot of this was that the delicate balance and months of work building trust with the other party was now more complicated and convoluted. Sadly, the attempts to rebuild and recover the process, and indeed it was a complex transaction-now made more so, were not successful and this potential merger failed. Was this failure caused solely by the board members actions? Probably not. It may have collapsed on its own weight, but we will never know. What we do know is that the other entity did complete a transaction with another party, one from outside of the marketplace. The advantages we sought and desired from this potential alignment were lost and have never been replaced.

Because of the complex health care environment, trustees often focus internally, ignoring community needs. It is human nature to try to make all problems simple so that they can succumb to a simple solution, so this is understandable, albeit ill-advised. This can be verified through periodic community assessments that may show a misalignment of the hospital with its community. Hospitals, in the end, are assets designed for the community and should be transforming into what is best for the people they have the responsibility to serve. This requires attention to the full continuum of care and not just to disease management. It demands focus on the value of services, rather than just its own volume and occupancy.

It is a red flag when we see board goals not paralleling the CEO's goals. Annual board self-evaluations, board education and job descriptions or desired competencies of the board are often absent. Changing regulations, payment models, payer mix, new entrants into the market and shifting inpatient volumes create a dynamic and complex market mix. This requires the best strategic and creative minds working in unison. Boards and management teams need to be aligned for the best possible outcomes.

## The Roles and Responsibilities of Excellent Boards

A board is responsible and accountable to the organization it is governing, ensuring that it is fulfilling its mission, living its values, and envisioning its future while always protecting its assets.

To do such, boards must act as a governing body that has designated roles and responsibilities, preferably written, that will best assure the hospital or health system will deliver efficient and effective care services. They must accept that the only system that will survive - and thrive - long term is one in which care is of the highest quality, safety, affordability, accessibility and is fully coordinated across the continuum. Boards must move from a socially driven "do not make waves" mentality to that of being the responsible party addressing the needs of the community.

More specifically, excellent boards embrace and monitor the following five roles and responsibilities:

1.  <u>Oversight of Performance</u> that ensures optimal clinical quality and safety with attention to service delivery, patient, employee and physician satisfaction and engagement is key. The board clearly has the responsibility to hire, evaluate and fire (as necessary) the CEO. Additionally, business literacy, including capital and operational budgets and regulatory compliance must be maintained. Finally, there must be an effort to provide community value, i.e., appropriate services, cost structure/affordability and accessibility in the continuum of care.

2.  <u>Outside-in thinking</u> can help to improve the strategic outputs. Special consideration must be given to monitoring of implementation and a pre-determined agreement on metrics of success. This is especially true given the board role in approving the strategic direction for the institution.

3.  <u>Generative thinking</u>, that is, future planning and envisioning the future eight to ten years out, rather than a focus only on what's at hand.

4.  <u>Self-assessment</u> and continuous education driven by the assessment process and community feedback.

5.  Board members must be fresh, creative and invigorated. Therefore, it's essential to have <u>term limits</u> and routinely <u>identify competent</u> and complementary new board and committee members.

Assuming accountability for these roles and responsibilities is no small task for the individual trustees and the board collectively. It requires the enhancement of knowledge and understanding of the present board members and the recruiting of new board members with the necessary experience and skills. Together, in concert with the CEO, they can guide the organization through the transformation changes to support a journey to excellence.

**Characteristics of Successful Boards**

In addition to the known and proven roles and responsibilities of successful boards, there are additional characteristics of highly effective boards that we have observed, experienced and endorsed.

<u>Size</u>: Boards can be too large or too small, and in both cases, can inhibit robust discussions and helpful interchanges. We have seen boards as large as fifty people. This is truly an unwieldy size. A meeting with this many people invites over-control by the board leadership to achieve some agenda or goal. When a meeting is constrained in such a way, few people are able to speak, question, comment, or even participate at all. A large board size and its self-limiting behaviors then invites members to send in their regrets for attendance at subsequent meetings. A too-large board is a prescription for governance failure caused by its own weight. Likewise, a board can be too small. Most boards have a minimum number of members identified as part of the incorporating documents…this is most often three people. While this may be the number accepted by the Secretary of State to legally conduct business, it is not a good governance practice to have so few. Why? Particularly for a healthcare institution, which is created to serve a community, it is important to get representation that reflects the best interests of that community; this means many more than three people. A board that is small is subject to cronyism, self-dealing, lack of governance accountability and a myopic sense of reality. So, just like the three bears

eating their porridge, boards should not be too large or too small, but just right. Research indicates that **the ideal board size** is between 12 and 15 members. (42)

Meeting Frequency: **Quarterly meetings are ideal**, with focused CEO communications to the board between sessions. Many boards meet monthly which is not always efficient. That said, the three of us, as leaders forming a new organization from a consolidation of two health systems, did have monthly board meetings for the first year and a half. We also had three Board strategic retreats during this same 18-month period. This worked because we needed the input of governance to the many, many consolidation considerations and policies we were considering and implementing. Circumstances and necessity drove the need for more meetings. As soon as it was deemed appropriate we went to quarterly meetings. The danger of meetings that are too frequent is that this pattern can turn boards into implementers and away from their true role as overseers. Quarterly meetings give management enough time to implement operational initiatives and begin to see the results of these efforts. These results are what boards should focus upon. Management should be allowed time for the complex operations challenges they face. Margin compression, new product offerings, quality issues, IT complexity and cyber-security, debt covenants and financial risks, physician alignment and contracts, turnover and recruitment, capital constraints, new technologies and the possible occurrence of a Black Swan is enough for any team. The distraction of preparing for a too frequent board meeting takes the leadership team away from the duties they are paid to perform. Especially if an organization is conducting quarterly meetings it is critical to allow enough time for the board to fully assess, dialogue and understand, and give direction to management. In our current consulting practice, we have seen boards that meet quarterly, but only over a long lunch or an evening meal. This is not sufficient. Meeting time should be adequate for a board to be able to function properly.

Personal Time: Board membership requires a significant **time commitment**. The unpaid or minimally compensated volunteer board members, need to read and study in advance of meetings. They should come to the table with as much knowledge as possible, and supplement such with additional information they acquire from the discussions in the room. Then, and only then, can they make informed decisions. When considering new additions to the board, many governing leaders tend to "recruit" these new members by emphasizing the positive, illustrating the importance of board service and playing up the sense of duty that a person should reflect upon in order to agree to join the board. They don't mention that board members are expected to come to meetings, to be on time and be prepared with advance reading. They don't mention that there is often a committee assignment (or two) that goes along with board membership and occasionally there are ad hoc obligations related to fund raising, community events and even attendance at educational sessions or seminars. These all, important and significant as they may be, require a personal time commitment by each member of the board, so the full obligation of participation on a board must be understood, accepted and lived out.

Decision Making: Regardless of how the board member got his or her position, the board member must realize that the responsibility is to **make and support decisions that benefit the good of the organization** as a whole. This means they must be open to hearing the recommendations of leadership, learning from the boards discussions and advance materials, and then supporting the consensus of the governing body. In this challenging environment, where solutions may require untried and unproven innovative approaches, decisions must be based on as much relevant and useful information as possible to minimize the risks that accompany any new undertaking. In the case of most health care organizations each member of the board is a fiduciary; that is, they are charged with upholding the highest standards of trust and duties of care and loyalty in which no conflict exists with carrying out these duties. A fiduciary is required to act always in the best interest and for the sole benefit of the one who places their trust in the board members lap. These traditional obligations for members of a governing board can be found in almost every management textbook ever written. In regards to decision making, a duty of a board member is to make the best decision on behalf of the organization. This must be done without consideration of any advantage or disadvantage to the individual board member. So, if done well and appropriately, the decision-making by the member is free of conflict and fully underscored with the relevant knowledge and facts necessary for a good and proper consideration. If the knowledge is lacking, if the facts are non-specific, it is the obligation of the member to seek clarification early on so a decision is not delayed unnecessarily. In short, board members need to show up, prepared and ready to work for the organizations mission and vision and do so within the framework of its values.

Fresh Thinking: You may have heard the phrase: 'don't work harder... work smarter'. Essentially this is what generative thinking is about. Think: generating new fresh ideas. Boards can follow all the rules of good governance behaviors, structure, time frames and still miss out on one of the most important aspects of being involved as a board, the collective power that can be unleashed when each member of the board brings to the table their experience, wisdom and intelligence. It is beyond setting strategic direction, it is beyond the duties of being a responsible fiduciary; it includes these things but it is about bringing the best questioning of assumptions and traditions and asking (in the context of the organizations own values) what are we really about? The status quo is no longer acceptable. This industry is moving too fast. There may be dinosaurs still in existence enjoying the fruits of stability and an unchallenged marketplace, but they will not be around for long. Change is always difficult, but if a true transformational journey is to occur, the **board members must lead the change** and not resist it. Setting board goals and expectations is an important outcome and which will ensure that the quality thinking from a dynamic board is not lost.

Composition of the board: Board members should commit to being health care and community focused, stewards of resources and strong team players. Board members are expected to utilize their talents to the fullest degree possible, strive to meld the different perspectives of the board members and leadership, be willing to compromise, and comfortable with robust discussions.

## Dynamic Health Care Board Checklist

The evolution of the board to an effective and excellent governing body, like all evolutions, requires well-defined transformational strategies that are embraced by all board members, old and new, as well as the CEO and the leadership team. Following are suggestions:

1. Develop and implement job descriptions for both the chair and members.
2. Perform board assessment, at least annually, to assure they are holding themselves accountable for best practices. Verify their successes from a multidisciplinary group they are serving, including leaders, physicians, and community members.
3. Keep the board competencies current and utilize them to drive the new board selection processes.
4. Implement a well-designed educational program for the trustees, covering all their roles and responsibilities and proven successful characteristics that they must embrace.
5. Consider, if not already present, putting physicians on the board to enhance the physician alignment strategy, so critical for an organization's successful transformation. This will undoubtedly require a clear conflict of interest policy, since the board will likely be addressing physician acquisitions and the like.
6. Appoint committees to assist the board. The committee structure reduces the work of the full board, brings forth recommendations that are usually based on more in-depth discussions than could be afforded at the regularly scheduled board meetings, and provides an opportunity to get prospective board members involved. If committees are utilized, however, they must have clear charters and agreed-upon roles and responsibilities, and report their recommendations to the board for final decision making.
7. Utilize input and recommendations from the CEO and the leadership team, to design, approve and implement a dashboard report containing outcome metrics to review at each meeting. This report should include the present performance measurements for all operational goals, as well as their end-of the-year expected levels.

If the expected levels are not being achieved, then performance improvement plans should be expected from leadership, explaining how the course correction will occur. This is the best way to develop a culture of accountability within the organization.

8. The board, in partnership with the CEO and the leadership team, should participate in annual strategic planning and then regularly hear reports and review data assuring that the plans are being followed and the strategies are being implemented. These strategies, at minimum, need to include those that will enhance physician integration, move to population management, encourage cooperation and collaborative efforts, and align incentives to the degree possible with all stakeholders, both internal and external.

9. Allot time to participate in generative discussions with leadership and community representatives. These will spur potential directions for the next eight to ten years. When this envisioned future looks like it is becoming reality, then the board and leadership will be much better prepared to incorporate their future learning into the organization's three-year rolling strategic plan.

In summary, excellent governance is key for an organization to be successful. The achievement of such is never an accident and must be intentional. It requires ongoing planning, focus and review. Based on our experience, it is clear excellent governance, when combined with excellent leadership and leadership teams, is the recipe for transformational work that will result in a bright future for any and all organizations. Excellent health care boards are dynamic entities that deliver better value in all they do.

# Chapter 8

# Competent Leadership

**"The real act of discovery consists not in finding new lands, but in seeing with new eyes." -- Marcel Proust**

**Leaders Must Make a Difference**

Implementing successful transformational strategies requires strong leaders who others will follow. This is challenging in an extremely complex health care environment. Effective leaders must have a set of competencies that not only includes their knowledge but also encompasses their abilities, skills, behaviors, and attitudes. Together these competencies become integrated to become their leadership style. Hence knowledge-driven leadership, once acceptable and adequate, has had to be transformed into a competency-driven model. This transformation is required both for the more traditional nonclinical administrative leaders and the increasing number of physician executives that are being added to the leadership teams, believing they will drive both the quality initiatives and the physician integration strategies.

What must not change is the definition of leadership. Although the specific words and sentence structure might vary, most articles and books on leadership define it as the ability to inspire the staff to do what is necessary to drive the organization to excellence. This requires that all stakeholders develop ownership in a shared mission, vision and values.

Successful leaders must drive the operational focus and performance outcomes while leading the strategic planning and the implementation of the supporting tactics. Finally, a leader must encourage visionary and innovative thinking. At the end of the day, leaders must make a difference, and to do that, they must always believe they can. There are, understandably with the complex challenges, many ways for leaders to fail, but perhaps one of the most important may be the failure of will.

## The Old Paradigm of Leadership

In the past, the main leadership style was hierarchy. The CEO was the boss. Senior executives and their managers often saw themselves as the boss's mini-bosses. So, the organization developed a controlled environment driven from the top down. Leadership education was not a high priority, and clarity of goals and expectations was often lacking. Negativity resulted in poor performance and was rarely balanced by rewards and recognition when things were going well. When decisions were made, they often resulted in win/lose situations that polarized and fragmented the leadership team.

CEOs often saw their major roles as external to the organization, spending significant time in advocacy and association activities, with little clarity on who was in charge while they were away. Financial risks were far less, thus, an absentee style of leadership was tolerated. CEOs of the past often led reactive rather than proactive processes, spending little time learning from their failures.

Many leaders were change averse and valued tradition over innovation. Maintaining peace was far more important than dealing with conflict, and, therefore, there was a low threshold for robust and candid discussions.

Because the old paradigm was different, the leadership requirement for success was different. It seems abundantly clear that the leaders of the past, who could or would not have participated in transformational action, would not be successful in this new healthcare environment.

## Leadership in the New Paradigm—the Transformational Leader

Taking "what is" and making it into "what it needs to become," may be the simplest way to express the road map for leadership for health care organizations now. Complex times demand transformational leadership. The new transformational leaders must combine knowledge with other competencies to deliver transformation. Among those ingredients are:

- vision, creativity and innovation
- high ethics and values, integrity and trust
- proven analytical and strategic planning and prioritizing know-how
- timely and smart decision making and problem solving
- strong verbal and written two-way communication
- team builder adroit in conflict management
- result-driven change agent

In addition, effective leaders must function and perform successfully in three different levels of the organization:

On the stage—assuring that operations, monitored by a balanced scorecard of best-practice metrics, are producing positive outcomes in clinical delivery, service levels and business measurements while enhancing their value to the community.

In the balcony—driving a strategic-planning process with well-defined tactics, designated responsible parties and appropriate timelines for completion.

In the clouds—leading visionary and innovating thinking while envisioning what the organization may look like in eight to ten years.

Given that physicians are the major drivers of cost and quality, they will be called on more and more to take on leadership responsibilities. Both physician and administrative leaders must become less hierarchical. Top-down, control-oriented leaders will not be able to drive transformation changes that guarantee sustainable success for the organization's journey into the future.

## The Risks of Transformational Leadership

There is significant agreement that leading health care today is probably one of the most challenging CEO roles (43), when compared to other industries. CEOs often find themselves in extremely risky positions, because of the transformation processes needed to be successful in this new paradigm. The CEO's goals and expectations are often not clearly defined, and frequent and candid performance evaluation discussions between the CEO and board chair are many times lacking. The finger is quickly pointed at the CEO when the performance metrics are not reached. This results in leaders feeling vulnerable and much more unsure of job security. Uncertainty and insecurity creates negative outcomes, which if not addressed could lead to a leadership vacuum. Consider the following:

1. The turnover rate among CEOs in the health care industry is nearly 20 percent, the highest it has ever been. (44) Although boards are forcing some of this turnover, a large portion is due to voluntary resignations submitted by CEOs who say they can no longer take the pressure, or it is no longer worth it. Most of these are well-credentialed health care administrators.

2. Early retirements are often occurring before appropriate succession plans can be put in place, resulting in leadership voids, which are most significant when organizations are challenged.

3. The trend is for hospitals and health systems to appoint CEOs with no prior health care experience. A recently published poll of 1,404 health provider organizations indicated that nearly two-thirds of CEOs hired in 2014 had little or no health care sector experience. Other poll findings reported:
   - The average tenure of a hospital CEO is under 3.5 years.
   - More than half (56 percent) of CEO exits are involuntary.
   - Nearly half of CFOs and COOs are terminated within nine months of a new CEO's hire, as well as 32 percent of marketing officers.
   - A high 87 percent of chief medical officers are replaced, most within two months, after a new CEO is appointed.

- Almost all (94 percent) of new CEOs without extensive hospital backgrounds indicate they do not believe health care expertise is needed for a management overhaul.
- Approximately nine in ten (89 percent) board members hiring outsiders agree that broad business operational expertise, singular vision, cost savings and the goodwill to the community are important. (45)

4. At the same time, we are aware of proposals that all health care sector CEOs should be physicians since <u>physician integration</u> is a critical success factor. (46) Physician resistance to change is well known. Physician leaders often have the best chance of convincing their medical colleagues to change their positions. Indeed, a number of successful health care organizations that have a long history of stability and growth—Mayo, Cleveland Clinic, and Geisinger Clinic as examples—have always had physician CEOs. There is no doubt that a good clinician can transition to become a good executive, but it is often not an easy road. Physician leaders must participate in learning opportunities to acquire the competencies necessary for leadership success. A good leader should be chosen, not because of his or her clinical background, but because of their demonstrated skill at leading. There are many physicians who can be, and are, excellent leaders.

The candidate pool of leaders to be considered for the growing number of vacancies must include a variety of backgrounds, such as clinical and other broad industry experience. Without expanding the pool to include different and new talent this may result in perpetuating a vicious cycle in more CEOs being forced to step down. It is easy to see how all of this may be the cause of the significant leadership vacuum at a time when perhaps the competent leader is the most important key to the organization's success.

## Strategies to Assure Effective Leadership

As in all positions, the greatest guarantee of a person being successful is to make sure the best person was selected for the job. Recruiting and hiring must be driven by a set of proven principles and steps, carried out in an orderly fashion. Based on the challenges the organization is facing, a clear set of performance goals should be written into the successful candidate's profile. This list should then drive the competencies that the leader must have to reach these goals. Once the competencies are identified, each candidate should be asked to put in writing and expand on verbally in the interviews clear "lived" examples of how they demonstrated these competencies in their prior positions. If they do not appear to have competency to the degree necessary, then the candidate should be able to present a convincing education process he or she will undertake to obtain that competency in an appropriate period of time.

Once hired, the CEO should have performance evaluations with the board chair, or a committee of the board for better continuity, and the CEO should do the same for his or her leadership team members, evaluating progress being made on reaching agreed-upon success metrics. At the bare minimum evaluation sessions, must be held annually.

If adequate progress is not being demonstrated, then a written performance improvement plan should be formulated, with clear deadlines for completion. Evaluations should be more frequent in a new leader's early tenure or when the performance is deemed unsatisfactory. It is most effective when feedback to the leader is supported by data gathered from a 360-degree survey of peers and superiors, including all board members in the case of the CEO. We are strong advocates for frequent feedback for the CEO.

The strategies outlined to assure successful leaders may seem obvious. However, successful leadership is not always the sole purview of the leader, it often depends on others and they have responsibilities as well. Consider a leader who may have to depart an organization; when one explores more fully why a specific leader was terminated, one often finds that neither the leader nor board had a clear understanding of the desired performance goals and expectations. Clear expectations need to be communicated both verbally and in writing. In the end, it is rare that the dismissed leader has full ownership of his leadership failure. True accountability can only be had when the performance goals are clearly articulated and agreed upon by all parties.

## Passion Breeds Success

Whether the staff is willing to follow the leader depends significantly on the passion of the leader. Passion is heard in the tone of the voice, seen in facial expressions, and broadcast by body language. It is embedded in the words that are spoken and written. When present, it will inspire others to follow, ultimately creating a passionate organization, a critical characteristic of a successful health care brand.

In addition, passion breeds enthusiasm, operational focus, accountability, and innovation, all critical success factors in any organization's culture and leadership team. Therefore, leaders must ignite their passion for their work. They should have, and exude, a positive outlook, regardless of the level of stress and challenges they face.

Many physician leaders and administrative leaders are expressing just the opposite, deciding to retire earlier than planned, and telling the younger generation that they should not pursue careers in health care. By enhancing the passions of the leadership team, this negativity can, it is hoped, be reduced and even eliminated. Passion is the place where the love of your work lives, and without it, the road map for change might prove too daunting.

## Developing Passion

All leaders need to believe that health care is a sacred ministry. Patients and family members come through the office or clinic doors entrusting their lives or the lives of their loved ones to a caregiver. This is perhaps the greatest responsibility for each and everyone working in health care today.

Leaders need to believe, in some way, that their work is a calling rather than just a job or a profession. People doing a job each day can do satisfactory work, and people who are professionals clearly can do meaningful work. Passion can be ignited when leaders stop and ask, as they are performing patient-centered activities, whether in their administrative offices, operating rooms, emergency departments, hospital rooms, or ambulatory settings, "Could this be one of the reasons I was put on this earth?" Regardless of the age, gender or role any leader has, the answer to this question should be a strong and resounding "yes." Knowing this ultimately gives the leader the ability to enthusiastically lead each day, in both good times and bad. Such enthusiasm will be contagious, creating, in turn, a large family of professional and passionate followers.

# Chapter 9

# Teamwork

**"Talent wins games, but teamwork and intelligence wins championships." -Michael Jordan**

## There Is No "I" In Team

This is a people paradox. There is little space today for the "I" in the leader's communications if the best administrative decisions are to be made and the best clinical outcomes are to be achieved. Even if it could be proven that one person is usually responsible for all the positive outcomes, the potential rise and fall of the organization driven by the performance of one individual would result in an intolerable enterprise risk. This would be especially dangerous in today's climate when CEO turnover is nearly 20 percent and more physicians are retiring early. (48)

Yet, it's not uncommon to hear a CEO, in response to pressure from the board, say, "This is what I have done positively." Unfortunately, this defensive attitude or belief that he or she alone did something positive emanates from leadership arrogance that can creep into one's behavior from having the top title and the highest salary, especially if the CEO sees his or her position as one of power and control. This type of response is seen both in health care organizations' administrative and physician leaders, maybe even more in the latter.

In the past, when the health care industry was facing less complex challenges, a strong leadership team was a luxury, great to have but not a critical success factor. Perhaps that is why these times were often populated by very powerful, controlling, hierarchical CEOs who catered to a physician-centric and volume-driven environment. Today, needed transformational strategies must shift the organization to an integrated population health and wellness care structure. This new model demands the collective expertise of all members of the leadership team to drive the outcomes that will enhance quality and safety, lower costs and increase accessibility.

When you ask the leaders of successful organizations today to what they attribute their success, they often respond it's the strength of their teams and the competencies of their people. No one person has all the answers. While in the past teaming might have been a luxury, today it is a necessity.

**Barriers to a Strong Team**

Even if some CEOs tout that they have a strong team model, the CEO or COO are often prescriptive and expect total compliance with their directions. This compliance is often a result of maintaining a high level of fear among the team members. To assure job security, team members remind themselves daily that their job is to carry out their boss's direction.

The recruiting process can stand in the way of having a cohesive and effective team. Many people are hired to do a specific job, usually encased in a longstanding organizational silo. These employees are taught that the most important person is the one they report up to, rather than who they work with laterally. This practice results in an organizational chart populated by strong solid lines rather than the dotted lines that signify a strong team focus.

In such a hierarchical environment, the expected performance outcomes are often immediate and have a short-term focus. This approach does not encourage the cross-service line building blocks formed by multidisciplinary groups of people, which are the foundation of a successful long-term transformational journey.

If forming cohesive and strong teams were easy, we would see them much more frequently. Therefore, the creation of such must be intentional. The role modeling, coaching, and mentoring, so critical to strong team formation, must be visible at all levels of the organization, as well as among board members. In our last organization, we initiated a system-wide mentoring program. We knew that to develop the bench strength we needed to go forward in a changing health industry we need to be intentional and committed. A thoughtful approach was necessary for success. Mentors themselves had to be identified, but also had to be schooled in what was a proper experience between mentor and mentee. We asked for progress reports from both parties. We asked mentees to work in teams together to identify opportunities for growth that could enhance their relationship with the assigned mentor. The final evaluation often resulted in a mentee 'graduating', so to speak, to an unofficial category of young talent. These folks, now so identified, were given additional opportunities to grow and succeed. Indeed, they were the future leaders who became part of our teams.

Success should not be given to, or accepted by, just the people at the top of the company. Rewards for effective teaming, even a simple "thank you," should be done frequently. This is another example of where mal-aligned incentives will ultimately lead to failure, whereas reward and recognition drive success. Dr. Tom had a lifelong habit of writing personal notes to people, most of them thank you notes or messages of congratulations and encouragement, daily. This was just part of his modus operandi. The importance of this was brought home once while he was in leadership at Johns Hopkins University Medical Center in Baltimore. At a retirement reception for one of the medical professors, a person who many years earlier had won a Nobel Prize. Dr. Tom had the opportunity to visit with this doctors' wife. She said something very meaningful about the importance of personal recognition. She shared that even though her husband had been recognized professionally his entire career for his many salutary accomplishments and for his extensive publications and contributions to medicine, which of course culminated in a Nobel Prize, it was Dr. Tom's personal note that was stuck on the refrigerator door in their kitchen. The note served as a daily reminder to each of them that someone cared. In the heart of each human there lies a need to connect to another…and this may be more important than money, notoriety or fame.

When teaming is not seen as a critical success factor, it is not built into job descriptions, yearly performance improvement discussions and plans. Without such, the achievement of a strong team has no accountability or recognition, and individual achievements continue to be the primary focus. Such is a red flag for failure.

## The Teaming Transformation

If, indeed, the answers to the complex challenges facing health care today require the collective thinking of groups of competent individuals working together in an integrated and collaborative fashion, then the formation of strong teams must become a transformational strategy.

Strong teams, like strong families, are grown rather than born. Individuals can learn the teaming skills, accepting the need to make sacrifices at times for the good of the whole. They learn how to listen well, and provide feedback in an understandable manner. Strong team members are willing to change their position if appropriate, and support the consensus of the group. In addition, healthy team players learn how to tolerate high anxiety, develop trustful relationships and have a loyalty to each other. They know, however, that this loyalty must not be to the level that prevents realistic discussions, complete honesty and sometimes agreements to disagree.

Strong teams understand the need to take risks, and do not tolerate finger pointing; they learn how to improve in a positive manner. Teams are also able to "garage sale" effectively, looking at what they are doing that no longer is necessary and then, more importantly, giving it up. Teams use this freedom to more effectively oversee daily operations and drive the strategic plans, and realize resulting growth.

Teams know that every decision they make is not perfect, or the right one. Therefore, they must be flexible and honest enough to admit their mistakes and incorporate plan 'B' into their journey. They must be resilient, remaining optimistic during difficult and challenging times. They may find themselves in a valley, or on a rough detour on their journey, but they must never lose sight of their final destination.

Finally, excellent teams are committed to lifelong learning, knowing that more change will always be on the horizon. As a result, they constantly are sharing informative articles, reviewing journals, studying environmental assessments and networking with others to learn about the latest trends and best practices.

## Maintaining Cohesive Teams

Even when there is a strong commitment for, and the successful implementation of, an effective cohesive team, maintaining such on an ongoing basis can prove difficult. There are many recurring staff behaviors that can weaken the team process. Most of these deal with "I".

The strong individual focus of administrators and physicians will rear its head periodically, causing the team effort to be less effective. When leaders have learned to function in a command and control mode, they will see teaming as potentially weakening their control, making the ability to command difficult. They must be reminded that the origin of their fears is understandable, but their fears must be overcome. Losing control equates to a loss of power and is seen by some leaders to parallel the degree of support for teaming. Hence, they believe strong teaming may cause them to lose their personal ability to influence the destiny of the organization. If such a person feels that their personal influence is lost they will then likely also have a loss of recognition as an individual. This could weaken one's self-esteem and is seen as a problem by some leaders. An individual-focused approach results in more individual accolades and recognitions. A less mature team player may ask silently or openly, "Who is going to get the credit for this successful outcome?" For these leaders, team recognition is not enough. It is important to remember that strong teams are made up of strong, confident individuals who know that playing together is far more successful than playing alone.

Knowing that being a team is an expectation, some leaders will support the team in a meeting but go back to the "I" mode when leaving the room.

This is a common problem and often hard to detect. This often comes as a result of a leader not supporting the consensus of the team. We know of a situation at an organization that had a member of the senior team who had a habit of questioning decisions that had had already been made previously by the entire team, including ones that they themselves had participated in. Certainly, every senior leader should be open to pushback and to reflection that may cause a reappraisal of a decision or even a new direction. As we said earlier there is no perfect decision. However, when a member of the team consistently revisits a decision, and here we are talking about 75% of the time, then there is a problem either with this person's ability to process information and reach a conclusion on a timely basis or there is a personal need to draw the attention of the group back to this individual in a controlling kind of way. Once this pattern became clear it was dealt with handily. Passive-aggressive behavior, if not addressed, can quickly deteriorate the team's effectiveness and credibility. It must be censured. Wrong decisions are inevitable but it takes a team approach to rectify the miscalculation. A weak team player is often quick to claim "teaming does not work" when the issue may or problem may have been caused by their own ineffectiveness. If this person's "blame-shifting" is allowed to fester, the strength of the team is undermined.

Traditionally, the human resource function has, as part of its overall role, individual hiring, evaluations, compensation and equitable benefits for all. HR departments are increasingly embracing new models that align incentives and a job descriptions with the organizations transformational strategies, including team rewards and recognitions. Some leaders believe that all in the workplace should be treated equally at all times. They believe in an egalitarian approach to work. Unfortunately for them this is not a characteristic of a successful team. Just as on a sports team, the coach might ask some more qualified members to appropriately take the lead. When this happens, the team members who feel they have been benched may cry "foul." On one occasion, due to a transition by a key operator and health system leader, we had to create an ad hoc team to address this person's duties and obligations. We formed this team from a subset of the existing senior leaders. Because this person's role had been critically important and significant the magnitude of the issues that this ad hoc team had to address were major. So, the profile of the ad hoc team, which included us and some others, also rose. This created some consternation among the senior team leaders who were not a part of the ad hoc operating team. How did we deal with this issue? In retrospect, probably not as well as we would have wished. We tried explanation, justification and rationalization. It did not work. So, even though this ad hoc team was working well, and, in fact, was making measurable improvements in managing several operational issues, we capitulated. Lesson learned, or should we say reinforced: when a pathway has been selected and it is bearing fruit, don't deviate simply because someone may have their feelings hurt.

Many leaders have only worked in a solid-line, vertically reporting structure. They may initially resist working in a dotted-line, matrix model. These people have difficulty when they are not sure who the team leader is, each and every moment, and they lack the flexibility to work in a horizontally oriented structure, which is a requirement for the integrated and coordinated transformational strategy to occur.

Teams that are made up of members who are accustomed to working at their own pace, which now must comport to the team's timeline for completion of the assigned task are like oil and water, they don't mix. Sadly, not every team member may have the skills, or desire, to accept the team's schedule. They become the weakest link and, if not dealt with, will pull the entire team down. Tolerance of mediocrity is a major leadership challenge and creates a barrier to achieving excellence.

Just as achieving excellence, although challenging, is much easier than sustaining excellence, sustaining a strong and effective team is more difficult then the initial implementation of one. The cohesiveness of the team must be continuously monitored, and if any of the anti-team behaviors becomes evident, it should be addressed and eliminated as quickly as possible. In the end, the strength of the CEO's team is more critical than his or her individual strength if a successful transformation is to be implemented and sustained.

## The Checklist for Competencies of Effective Teams

Just as we noted, earlier, that successful leaders have individual competencies, successful teams have team competencies. The understanding and development of these are part of a critical process that must be undertaken on the transformational journey. The organization's mission, vision and values are the foundation for effective teams. Strong teams can be built by having an inherent trust of each other's intentions. They must embrace known success competencies, and educate each team member on how these should be grown and incorporated into their daily behaviors and performance.

<u>Open communication and trust.</u> Strong communications instill, a sense of connectivity. Each member must be fully informed of all aspects of any project, whether operational or strategic, good or bad. The entire team must be comfortable with openly sharing ideas, and-in the midst of open candid discussions also know and practice total respect for confidentiality. Where trust exists, there is a deep-rooted faith and reliance on all members. This can foster acceptance of constructive criticism that, in turn, builds a more successful outcome for the team.

<u>Embracing stretch goals.</u> Team goals should exceed the goals of the individual. Team pride is buoyed when stretch goals are met or surpassed.

<u>Entrepreneurialism and innovation.</u> Team members help each other explore new ideas.

- Time to develop new ideas is scheduled, and not labeled as non-revenue producing time.
- Reflection on ideas is encouraged, to advance the transformational vision of the company.
- Team members are empowered, and encouraged, to take risks and innovative approaches.

Robust discussion and debate.

- Decisions should be formulated, and implemented, after careful discussion of all the potential pros and cons, even in times of uncertainty.
- Punitive Monday morning quarterbacking should not be tolerated. Rather, team members constructively discuss and challenge one another's ideas and approaches.
- Team members are open to listening to other team members' perspectives, and are open to changing their positions after hearing other approaches.
- Team members support the team's consensus to all audiences, internal and external.

Comfort with conflict and divergence of ideas.

- Team members experience personal tension comfortably.
- Team members recognize that conflict is a necessary part of successful team discussions.
- Team members try to transmit a friendly, easy going and relaxed character into their workplace and meetings.

Results driven with recognition.

- Learning is done through debriefing sessions.
- Successes are celebrated, even incremental victories.
- A high level of accountability for predetermined metrics of success is strongly embraced and supported for every project or task.

Complementary.

- Teams are created with members offering complementary skills.
- The value of the entire team is greater than the value of the sum of each of the team members. One plus one should equal eleven.

## Monitoring Team Competencies

Just as we suggested for excellence in governance, periodic evaluations of competencies are essential for all health system management teams. This assessment should begin with a group discussion by the team about which competencies they believe are working effectively, and those that they feel are weaker and need attention. Then each team member should be asked to rank each competency on a scale of one to ten. Next, individual ratings are aggregated to create team ratings. These, in turn, permit the competencies to be ranked from best to worst. Those receiving the lowest scores, perhaps six or below, should have a task force assigned to them to determine steps for improving that competency. This process, or one like it, will assure that the effectiveness is never taken for granted. Complacency fosters a belief that all is going well when perhaps it is not. Periodic monitoring and reassessment are ways to bar complacency from replacing one of the other team competencies.

Highly functional teams are critical for an organization's transformational journey to be successful. The competencies and attributes of such teams can be identified, taught, and implemented. By making team building an intentional strategy and monitoring it on a regular basis, sustainability of cohesive and effective teams should be possible, thus contributing to the organizational goals.

Some have often thought health care would be so much better if, rather than golf, an individually oriented sport, being the favorite pastime of administrative and physician leaders, they should all be playing basketball, soccer or football in their spare time. These sports require a strong understanding of what teaming is all about, and demand that it be in place every moment of the game.

Working well together is easy to say, but making it a reality requires not only an acceptance of the importance of the team approach but also a commitment to focus continuously on strategies to improve the team's functionality.

# Chapter 10

# Effective and Efficient

**"Impossible is just a big word thrown around by small men who find it easier to live in the world they've been given than to explore the power they have to change it. Impossible is potential. Impossible is temporary. Impossible is nothing." -- Muhammad Ali**

**Finding, and Following, the Way**

Operational effectiveness is neither a new nor narrow topic. Business process reengineering, Six Sigma, Lean, Toyota production system, outsourcing, and total quality management are just a few of the many concepts that have been used by organizations to improve operational effectiveness in the new millennium.

Many books with "Way" in the title, such as "The Toyota Way," "The Wal-Mart Way," "The Southwest Airlines Way," "The Samsung Way," "Jack Welch and the GE Way," "The Caterpillar Way," and "The Cleveland Clinic Way," document companies having superior operational effectiveness. Given the vast research and documentation of what makes organizations successful, why does health care seemingly lag in this area, and how will it radically improve? Before we answer this question, let's review what operational excellence is.

In many instances, operational excellence is initially identifiable by an organization's financial success. In other instances, it's identifiable by an organization's brand recognition. In other circumstances, it has to do with high-quality service delivery, that is: high quality and best of breed performance for procedural behavior as well as exceeding customers expectations. In whatever manner, operational excellence is identified, providing patients/customers with a solution to a need that is superior to the competitions is crucial. This creates revenue and, along with a very efficient cost structure, operating income. Being able to perform this act over a long period results in operational excellence. This is where the proverbial rubber meets the road. Not surprisingly, this isn't breakthrough thinking as authors like Peters and Waterman found in writing <u>In Search of Excellence</u> more than 30 years ago, (49) Jim Collins found similar results that he chronicled in <u>Good to Great</u>. (50) There are identifiable operational characteristics that contribute to organizations' success and longevity. Operational excellence consists of many moving parts that require constant attention and care to ensure both financial results and patient/customer satisfaction.

As previously discussed, disruptive factors are impacting health care from many different directions. At the writing of this book, many of these changes are in early stages, and the full impact is yet unpredictable. We are confident, however, in conveying a sense of urgency in regards to the need for a significantly higher level of operational performance for all health care providers in the future. Operational excellence is a precursor for successful transformation initiatives, indeed, it is a requirement. Present variables that contribute to the uncertainty are the pace employers will continue to incentivize employees to make better health care choices, the government's cost-reduction efforts, new providers offering lower prices because of lower operating costs, and employers opting out of providing health care benefits and placing employees in the health care exchanges. Much remains to be discovered.

With many hospital providers being tax-exempt organizations, appropriate financial goals are often determined by governing boards and not the vagaries of Wall Street. Being credit worthy, that is, getting an 'AA' rating from a financial analyst is, however, a significant marker for a successful not-for-profit organization. Presently, some organizations are setting financial objectives that would enable the organization to either break even, or even make a margin, at Medicare payment rates. Both government payers and employers are implementing programs to curb health care cost increases to be more in line with general inflation. Whether internally or externally generated, real improvement in operational performance is necessary to adapt to the changes.

## The Culture of Success

Earlier, we addressed the importance of the brand, and culture. The significant advantage of many successful organizations is an enduring culture of success. This means the organizational culture was set in place at the very beginning of the organization's existence. In many cases, it was the founder's DNA. This is the starting point. Is the organization's culture supportive of operational excellence? Does the organization's culture match the demands the organization is facing? An organization's culture provides the atmosphere in which everything else gets done. Will the organization's culture support change or resist change? The culture determines whether people will be compliant or committed to the organizational vision and goals. One measure of a culture that is improving, or as we say, is on the rise, is whether or not more and more associates can quote and live out the stated mission and vision. The challenge culture presents is most executives have little experience dealing with the concept.

Two notable executives that directly took on organizations with long, deeply embedded cultures were Jack Welch at General Electric and Louis Gerstner at IBM. Welch's tactics earned him the nickname of "neutron Jack." Early in Gerstner's tenure at IBM, the business press criticized him for his lack of focus. In Gerstner's book, <u>Who Says Elephants Can't Dance? Inside IBM's Historic Turnaround</u>, he discusses the important role culture plays in any organization. (51)

For many leaders, organizational culture development is just another passing management fad. Compared to strategy development, reengineering, financial planning, lean implementation, or marketing deployment, working on culture can feel like molding Jell-O. Yet, all successful organizations have strong cultures. The cultures reinforce and hold constant the practices that enable companies to be successful. Unfortunately, as the business environment changes, these same cultures then become the obstacles to change and threaten the organization's future. Instead of addressing the culture, leaders and managers resort to implementing more hierarchy and more bureaucracy to instill control to get things done. As Jim Collins pointed out in his book, <u>Good to Great—Why Some Companies Make the Leap ... and Others Don't</u>, (52) cultures can be enablers of successful results or can create bureaucratic environments that stifle people's desire to be outstanding.

Here's the tricky part. There is an ever-increasing abundance of tools available to make health care organizations more efficient, from productivity measurement tools to logistical deployment tools. Billions of dollars have been spent on electronic medical records. Billions more are going to be spent attempting to implement processes to make hospitals more operationally efficient. For a variety of reasons, the culture of many health care organizations is hierarchical, bureaucratic and command and control oriented. Thus, almost by intent operational change becomes difficult. Transformational change is impossible. During times when the status quo is sufficient, these organizational structures are effective in gaining compliance and conformity. When an industry wide change like shifting from fee for service healthcare to a value-based model occurs, rigid cultures become problematic. As innovation, creativity, speed and adaptability become the new determinants of success, leaders can find themselves trapped by the culture of the organization. Before investing any resources in tools, technology or education, stop and perform an assessment of the organization's culture. Without an understanding of the organization's culture, much time and resources can be wasted. Many leaders have attempted to implement change within cultures of mediocrity and have discovered the culture defeats whatever management change initiative is attempted. A culture of excellence is foundational.

## High Performing Teams and Individuals

The second step in the operational effectiveness journey is people. The challenge today's organization must contend with is creating both the high-performing team and the high-performing individual. Successful organizations are developing processes and structures that enable both. Historically, law firms, accounting firms, engineering firms, consulting firms, investment banks, technology companies have been recognized for their ability to recruit the best and the brightest from our nation's best colleges and universities. These colleges and universities have similarly developed rigorous screening processes to attract the best and brightest high school graduates as their enrollees. As global-competition has increased competition for talent in every business, talent recruitment and retention have become extremely important.

After assessing the organization's culture, evaluate the organization's workforce. Most hospital organizations are in the early stages of developing the necessary processes to sustain world class workforces. While many jobs once only based in hospitals are now available in a variety of ambulatory or standalone delivery sites. This added competitive pressure has made the recruitment of high quality medical personnel even more challenging.

The evidence remains there is a very high probability that a hospital patient during the winter months is going to be cared for by several agency nurses because of nursing shortages. While a generally accepted practice in healthcare, is this really providing a patient with the highest quality of care? Imagine boarding an airplane and being greeted at the door not by the normally attired pilot of the airlines but a generically uniformed individual. Then during the pilot's greeting and announcements she lets everyone know she's from The Acme Pilot Agency and is filling in for the day.

In more extreme situations rural hospitals are closing because of an inability to recruit people. At the same time, quality demands are accelerating and adding higher expectations to every healthcare professionals' responsibilities.

As health care has grown in to a three trillion-dollar industry, there are growing similarities between other professional service firms and technology companies in terms of success and talent. The big business of hospital leadership has been recognized with million dollar CEOS being routine. In addition, hospitals have also become large employers of physicians. Thus, potentially changing the physician/organization relationship. Nursing compensation in some areas has exceeded the $100 thousand level and is rapidly approaching that level in most areas. For some key nursing positions, shortages have turned nurses willing to travel in to free agents earning more than $200 thousand a year. These circumstances are dramatically changing the workforce dynamics of the traditional hospital. Therefore, the human resource department needs to be adapting very rapidly to provide the support necessary to cope with all the changes.

If these thoughts seem too unrealistic, remember a significant percentage of hospital workers are either directly or tangentially responsible for the well-being of the patients. In an environment of accelerating quality expectations, greater outcome transparency and reimbursement based upon value equations, every hospital workers' role is going to undergo dramatic change. In this ultra-competitive environment, attracting the best and brightest might mean the difference between staying in business or going out of business. Think about your hospital's hiring process in this context. In December 2013, Southwest Airlines had 10,000 job applications for 750 flight attendant positions…not for the year, in approximately 2 hours. While this might sound extraordinary, Southwest typically receives approximately 150,000 applications annually for about 4,000 jobs. (53) Is your hospital attracting this type of interest in posted positions? If not, better figure out why?

In most hospital organizations, one will find some sort of platitude espousing the importance of the organization's workers. Unfortunately, our experience is that in many cases this is more espoused that actualized. Hospitals are being challenged on two new fronts as this book is being written. Value and quality. This is going to place added pressure on human resource departments to be very strategic on making contributions to these efforts. The good news is there is a vast body of information about what

Google, Apple, Toyota, Southwest Airlines and other successful companies have been doing to close the gap between what's espoused regarding how workers are treated and how they are treated and enable to be outstanding contributors.

**Process Improvement**

Total quality management, continuous quality improvement, quality function deployment, total quality control are just a few of the improvement process labels that emerged in the 1980s as United States manufacturing companies were forced to come to grips with the invasion of better-quality Japanese products. In 1986, Motorola developed a set of process improvement tools called Six Sigma. In 1987, Congress established the Malcolm Baldrige National Quality Award to recognize quality achievements of U.S. companies. In the early 1990s, the world was introduced to the Toyota production system and the concept of "lean production." Over time, a significant body of research and implementation of quality improvement processes has occurred in a variety of industries. For different reasons, health care is not one of them.

Creating sustainable operational excellence without some form of process improvement system is highly unlikely. We can't explain why health care has been so resistant to the various process improvement tools. At Royer Maddox Herron Advisors, we have suggested there are professional ideological conflicts that exist. We have speculated, even though nursing schools are beginning to adopt Quality and safety Education for Nurses (QSEN) that some nursing schools avoid the subject and the result is that their graduate nurses have no interest in, or understanding of, process improvement concepts. In looking at the curriculum of a major university's master's program in hospital administration, we found two courses on process improvement. (54) Looking at the academic backgrounds of most leaders, or key decision makers in health care organizations, they've had very little exposure to process improvement concepts or tools during their academic training. We conclude that the process improvement sophistication found in manufacturing organizations is rarely found in health care organizations. Where it does exist, it is most likely the result of a chief executive officer's mandate. This is the reality. Unless you are fortunate to be working in an organization that has some type of improvement process agenda, starting from scratch is a monumentally difficult process. If you're not a CEO and don't have your CEO's 110 percent support in starting this effort, we suggest working on your resume simultaneously.

Here's one widely publicized example of what happens in a hospital when processes break down. On September 25, 2014, Thomas Eric Duncan presented himself to a hospital emergency room for treatment. He explained he had recently returned from Liberia, Africa, but had not been exposed to anyone having Ebola. On September 28, he returned to the hospital by ambulance, now with Ebola-like symptoms. After a two-day delay, his blood work was sent to the Centers for Disease Control to be tested for Ebola, and results came back positive. Unfortunately, Duncan did not survive. In addition, two of the nurses involved in Duncan's care also contracted the Ebola virus. (55) Aside from the tragedy of the patient's death, other events created a national media firestorm of questions and finger pointing regarding the procedures that contributed to these results. This illustrates the power of context and a real life-and-death story to get people's attention. Two things make Ebola frightening. It's contagious, and it has a high mortality factor. That makes it attention grabbing for media coverage. Fortunately or unfortunately, depending upon your perspective, when processes in a hospital break down, it's not unusual for mortality risks to increase, but the amount of publicity those events receive is usually very low.

Another example, a bit less dramatic than the Ebola case described above, happened in one of our hospitals and caused us to rethink what we could do to help a patient. Almost all hospitals keep statistics on their daily activities; this documentation is often required for billing purposes. During an annual operational review of these statistics in one of our Emergency Rooms it was discovered that three patients had visited the emergency room over 200 times in one calendar year. In fact, one of these patients had visited the ER 366 times; an average of once a day for the entire year. Clearly these patients needed something other than emergency care. The patient with the most visits did not live in the city supported by our hospital, but in a rural area nearby, so she had to make an extra effort by traveling some distance to visit the ER. If we had not analyzed statistics, if we were not willing to delve deeper into processes to understand some underlying issues, these-as well as other patients-may have continued to misuse the emergency services provided by our hospital. After a careful chart and record review that was followed by personal interviews with these and other patients it became clear that these people, most of them were suffering from a chronic (but totally manageable) condition, needed something more than a clinical intervention. In short, they were coming to the ER for reassurance, for kindness, for emotional attention. The physical condition was the excuse to present to the ER staff. We examined many things. Were the protocols and processes at issue in the ER? No. Were the processes of the hospital, the billing department or the social service workers or something else at issue? No. Could we have made more appropriate referrals? We did make correct referrals, but the receiving professionals discharged the patients appropriately. Our solution to fix a misuse and overuse of an expensive clinical service was to start a new program we called the Community Health Worker (CHWs). These were not public health workers nor were they social workers nor were they clinicians. At our expense, we trained qualified and willing persons to serve their neighborhoods and rural communities in a holistic way. We trained them to understand the signs for serious issues, but we also asked them to undertake home visits and family visits and become a community resource. The CHWs became a key part of the community. They relieved stress for those needing it, they counseled the correct action to pursue if this was merited, they became a liaison for the professional clinicians and, as an unintended but beneficial consequence for the hospital, they strengthened its brand and reputation in the communities served. This entirely new service was a win-win. It helped the emergency room become more efficient and freed up space for truly serious cases. It also helped people by addressing their needs, unspoken and non-clinical, but important needs for them. It came about because of an audit looking at process statistics, and it was a good outcome...a true process improvement.

Resistance to improvement in health care may be partially attributed to process failure. In cases like those involving high-profile individuals where media scrutiny requires further examination of the underlying circumstances, organizations are forced to evaluate processes and procedures and make changes. Unfortunately, that's not always the case. On the Centers for Disease Control website is a discussion and link to a 2011 New England Journal of Medicine article regarding hospital-acquired infections. (56) Per the report, approximately 75,000 people died directly or indirectly from a hospital-acquired infection. Unlike a single Ebola case, this circumstance does not get the media attention, and therefore doesn't get the same level of process improvement. In every health care organization, there exist circumstances and context for initiating and applying process improvement tools. These opportunities need more research and understanding because if the lack of quality becomes a newspaper story publicizing mortality issues or other patient care issues, the increased visibility translates to negative notoriety—not something boards and management desire.

# Chapter 11

# Lifelong Learning

**"Learning Is Not a Product of Schooling but the Lifelong Attempt to Acquire it." --Albert Einstein**

It is extremely possible that in all our lives, there was a time, particularly after graduation from high school, college or graduate school; we felt we learned everything we needed to know. We were sure our brains were as full as possible with knowledge, leaving no room for additional learning. However wrong that thinking is in our personal or professional careers, it is particularly dangerous for leaders and governance boards in health care.

Health care is driven by new technologies, innovative research and evidence-based medicine -- all drivers for change. These rapidly occurring changes foster medical advances that result in higher quality and safer outcomes for the patients. Acquisition of knowledge and skills, and accepting change as a good thing, are key ingredients for leadership teams and board members. Implementing a commitment to lifelong learning is essential for leading transformation strategies that will help assure the long-term viability of the organization.

To assure that all staff delivers the most up-to-date administrative and clinical processes and procedures, this lifelong learning journey cannot be left to chance. It must not be erratic, but rather intentional and continuous. Formal processes should be identified and documented to hold all accountable for replacing what is ineffective, inefficient, and outdated with new, proven best practices that result in better outcomes. If we accept this commitment, we should never find ourselves pining for "the good old days." In reality, as we look back, they were not so good. Using the best techniques and knowledge available 20 years ago, we still were unable to save some of our patients, and even if they survived, we caused them unavoidable harmful side effects. Status quo is never acceptable in the health care delivery process.

## Implementation Has Gotten More Difficult

If we were totally honest, those of us who were in health care leadership in the 1980s and 1990s would say that leading our organizations then was significantly easier than the subsequent decades. Medicare and Medicaid reimbursement, fewer governmental regulations, less transparency, a dearth of accurate outcome data, and cost based reimbursement for inpatient stays all contributed to an industry that in some cases ran on autopilot. Leaders rarely, if ever, asked themselves and their team's essential questions that lead to successful implementation of transformational strategies:

1. Do we have the competencies required to be great leaders at this moment in time?
2. What significant changes are occurring that will require new competencies and skill sets?
3. How do we gain these new competencies?

It is only when an organization and its leaders ask these questions, and answer them honestly, that the board and CEO will make the necessary commitment to leadership development. This is often done by implementing an organizational development function within the Human Resources department. This leadership education must include both administrative and clinical leaders, including physicians, since the right solutions must address both the clinical and financial outcomes the services deliver.

As obvious as it is that continuous leadership development is a critical success factor, this was not always the case. Enhancing revenues was the major avenue taken to correct an organization's woes. This led to a significant emphasis on maximizing cost-based "reimbursement", with the effect of artificially inflating our costs. This unfortunately minimized our understanding of the relationship between our costs and our charges, which continues to plague the health care industry and would be a deathblow for any other company in today's environment.

In addition to the bottom line and days in cash, organizational success was rarely equated with the competencies of its people but rather with the size of the company, the number of buildings, the number of beds, and the latest technologies. People power was rarely seen as an important asset. In addition, holding the leaders and their staffs accountable for undertaking continuous clinical or administrative education was rarely documented as a requirement to work in the organization. Consequently, this requirement was absent in the annual review process, if in fact, that process was even carried out.

During these less complex and challenging times, staff members were often hired to do a job based on their educational degree, knowledge-driven credentials, and prior on-the-job training. "How do you adapt to change?" and "How do you remain current?" are two critical questions for new hires that were rarely asked in the past. In addition, coaching and mentoring by the older, more mature, and capable leaders were rarely seen as a critical part of their workday.

The most effective leaders in health care have been trained by the 70-20-10 percent rule. That is, 70 percent of their training came from on-the-job experiences with team members, 20 percent from coaching and mentoring, and 10 percent from educational courses and preparation. Leaders are molded by their role models and experience. If the competencies of their role models were not kept current, then those who looked up to them for guidance were undoubtedly not getting the best that there was to get. Much less being on the cutting edge they received dull and worn out modeling. They did not develop the necessary leadership skills to move an organization to where it needed to be.

Unfortunately, both in the past and present, leadership arrogance stands in the way of honest self-assessment. Some leaders think they are far better than their outcomes would indicate. This lack of true and data-driven insight creates a major barrier for leaders. They must embrace self-improvement processes and a strong commitment to continuous learning. Leadership arrogance leads people to believe they have it all, and have nothing to learn. Such leaders do most of the talking and very little listening. Their leadership style is command and control versus nonhierarchical. They are poor role models and are inadequate to lead today when adapting and leading change is the highest priority.

## Transformational Leadership Is Evolving

Fortunately, there are successful leaders today who are continuously developing the competencies to be effective transformational leaders. They recognize that well-trained, highly educated, broadly competent, and continuously improving individuals are required in their organizations to assure stability and growth potentials. They also know that where we have the right people we usually have the right outcomes. Just as important, they know that the opposite is also true: unprepared people drive inadequate results. They know that the right facilities and technologies are important, but that even without these, the right people will find ways to make it all work.

Organizational development programs, as mentioned in the previous chapter, have become an understandably high priority on the list of transformational strategies. By recognizing the need to be continuously updated, leaders are less likely to succumb to dangerous leadership arrogance. They, in turn, accept that being highly educated is not enough, and they must develop the necessary competencies to address and solve evolving challenges they face. They know that updating their professional learning toolbox on a regular basis is a necessity in order to guide their organization on their transformational journey to excellence.

## Barriers to Implementing Continuous Learning Opportunities

Nothing comes free. By encouraging and supporting the development of effective educational programs to keep the board, leaders, physicians and staff competent, one is creating a line item of expenses in what is probably an already challenging budget. Unfortunately, such items have been labeled, as non-revenue producing expenses. In challenging times when profitability is difficult to achieve, and raising the revenue line is almost impossible, non-revenue producing expenses are often the first cuts to be made to balance the budget. This is a huge mistake. It is understandable for leaders, in stressful times, to seek expense reductions. Their thinking may look like this scenario, one that we admit we have been pulled into: Setting up, teaching in and monitoring the effectiveness of continuing educational programs takes staff time and energy. And, compounding this commitment, another ramification of meaningful educational experiences is that the organization may be building more competent leaders than will be able to advance within their organization. Consequently, some good people doing good things will decide to seek new opportunities elsewhere. Unless the CEO believes that nurturing leaders is advancing the greater good, he or she might see their departures as a failure and a waste of time and money. If this happens, educational and developmental programs are sadly on the chopping block.

## Building a Lifelong Learning Environment

**Determining openness to change is key.** Examples of developing significant and successful change processes is a predictor of comfort with change. Such competencies must be identified to spearhead organizational transformational processes.

**Developing teamwork** should be incorporated into institutional educational programs. Across the board, team players must value continuous learning to be prepared to lead the next change coming down the road as their journey to excellence continues.

**Role modeling** is an important component of lifelong learning. Leaders must allocate a significant portion of their time to coaching and mentoring the present and future leaders in the organization.

A commitment to lifelong learning should be rewarded, either with compensation or very visible **recognition programs**. These recognitions will go a long way to keep these critical transformational leaders energized and focused on today's mission and tomorrow's vision.

Through continuous education, both formal and informal, **internal talent pools** will constantly develop. The people in these pools will eagerly accept the accountability for achieving positive outcomes, knowing that they may undertake innovative ideas and that the risks associated with such will be tolerated.

Successful leaders must be committed to lifelong learning. For many years one of our dedicated staff had a poster in her office that showed a picture of the earth taken from outer space with a caption that read "Learners Shall Inherit the Earth." Far from being a crass take off from one of the Beatitudes found in the Book of Matthew ("Blessed are the meek for they shall inherit the earth." Mt 5:5), and far from the common understanding of the word meek, which today most people define as weak, unassuming, lacking courage or timid, the understanding of the word meek in Biblical times was 'Power Under Control'; we believe that this is a great way to frame leadership today as well. Perhaps we all should be more meek. Leaders who are also learners, who have power but are under control, realize that the world around them is in a constant state of change, of evolution, of dynamic tension. Leaders were once students in school, in graduate courses and probably were mentored well by earlier leaders in their career; but what they learned then is not sufficient for a new environment. New learning must become a constant in everyone's career. There are myriad ways to "keep up." Commonly, leaders attend conferences and courses and are also readers of new material. We endorse these many approaches to learning, but candidly, we also feel that leaders should step out of their box and push themselves in creative ways. So, we strongly recommend that leaders should seek out peer learning groups.

Some of these become golf outings so it is good to pick wisely. Peer group learning can provide a forum for learning and testing one's notions in an environment that requires vulnerability, offers peer pressure and stimulates thinking in an egalitarian environment; all something that leaders need to be exposed to if they are going to live into the word "meek." We also recommend that all leaders, management and governance, read something regularly that they would never think to read about. For example, if a news magazine is part of one's typical casual reading, then pick up a magazine about religion or landscaping or flying or sailing. Choose something totally different then one's typical pattern. Begin with a magazine to stretch the mind a bit and then graduate to books. If management books are typically part of your reading material, go pick up a volume on Shakespeare's best plays, or a novel or a book on philosophy. Learning is about expanding horizons, it is about being open, it is about growth. Never stop seeking. Become a 'meek learner.'

# Chapter 12

## Envisioning the Future

**"The task is, not so much to see what no one has yet seen; but to think what nobody has yet thought, about that which everybody sees."—Erwin Schrodinger**

### Driver of Change

Peter's aunt Virginia, a fifth-grade school teacher for decades in California, used to sell encyclopedias during the summer. It was a great job for a schoolteacher. Every parent wanted to provide a readily available resource for their children. Aunt Virginia was a great teacher and well loved by her students and fellow teachers. She was no dummy, because every year she had a new set of customers who had gotten to know her, trust her and value her advice and counsel. While it was good business, it was also a great service. Those encyclopedias were cherished, and remained, in peoples' homes for decades.

What happened to all the encyclopedias that occupied our family bookshelves? (57) It is easy to say that a new market competitor came in and stole the business. However, there were competitors in the reference book space already, and they duked it out every summer with their respective armies of teacher-salespeople. So, what was the issue? It was a failure on the part of the encyclopedia companies to be aware of the true drivers for their customers. An encyclopedia was not just another book; it filled a specific purpose for a buyer. In this case, it was more than the information and content, it was about accessing this easily and at home. What the companies were really providing was convenience at home to the same information that someone could get at the local community library.

As our world has evolved, there is a new variation on access…the Internet through personal computers and mobile devices. Nowadays, the world's information is easily accessible. Moreover, it's updated every day, and doesn't take up yards of space in your living room or den. Instead of scanning through hundreds of pages to find what you're looking for, the search engine does all the work for you. Free. Aunt Virginia could never have imagined a world in which research was done with a click of a mouse, or from a tiny telephone. Change happens…constantly. Be ready.

**The First Criteria for Addressing the Future: Awareness**

No one can predict the future. We humans have lost much of what our fellow creatures in the animal kingdom have maintained—an intuitive sense of the world around us. This sense enables them to avoid danger, to seek shelter before a storm, to find a mate, to adapt in order to access life sustaining water and food. Since our intuitive sense has been compromised or sublimated over the last ten thousand years, we must substitute its value with the something that our fellow creatures in the animal kingdom do not have—imagination. This is easier said then done, but known and proven imaginative techniques, when properly applied, help us to envision the future. If we can imagine it, we can be prepared for it and, better yet, in many cases we can even influence its outcome.

What is the history lesson with the encyclopedia business and how do we apply it to the future? As Polonius said in Shakespeare's play Hamlet, "To thine own self be true." This means total awareness, unadulterated and unwashed. If we do not really know who we are, know where we are, or know how we are viewed by others, we risk not being a part of the future. Knowing our current reality allows us to understand the threats that can undo us. The business models of the encyclopedia publishers was based on competing with the best quality of information, the expertise of their sales force and establishing price points at which a dutiful parent could buy. While these elements were important they missed the fundamental driver. Know thy self…and thy customer. This is not easy, but it is a necessary precondition for sustainability and adaptability and becoming a part of the future.

## The Second Criteria for Addressing the Future: Courage

Among many students in basic training, special forces and the Navy SEALS, situational awareness was a mantra pounded into their skulls. We cannot achieve excellence if we are only focusing on what the day brings. Maintaining 20/20 oversight and scrutiny of the past, present and future is crucial, especially in this changing health care world.

Royer Maddox Herron Advisors evolved from many years of Tom Royer, Peter Maddox and Jay Herron working together for a large health care system. Our prior organization came about from a consolidation of two large regional health systems that formed a multi-billion dollar system in several states. The genesis of this was to strengthen both of the respective health ministries of two separate Catholic congregations. By forming one larger system there would be great synergies from a common historical perspective and legacy, leverage in purchasing and expense control and a more significant presence for the faith-based orientation to health and hospital care. The resulting aggregation of services, people, policies, procedures, and practices was time consuming, and required an immense amount of focus.

The prior organizations had existed for more than 130 years each. There was substantial history and identity for each of the health systems. We needed to create a new culture, a new orientation to who we now were. We needed to go forward together, and we needed to do this quickly. It did not help that we had tremendous challenges on the financial side to include a first year multi-million dollar loss in net income and substantial millions of dollars in capital expenses. With this as a formidable backdrop, but with the aura of the honeymoon still in place, the senior management team proposed to the Board of Directors that we undertake a study of the future to prepare this new organization for a changing world. The board may not have fully appreciated what it had approved, but approved it was and we were off and running on a process which would inform and form our organization in a way no other could.

"What the _____ do you think you are doing? And where in the world are we going?" These were words spoken to us by the Chair of the Board at the end of the first day of our Futures Task Force retreat. The question was a fearful one. Here we were a newly formed organization needing to do so many operational things to accomplish the intent of the consolidation. It was a time of high anxiety. Our margins were non-existent and the financial forecast was challenging. We had bondholders to please, objectives to meet and more tangible things to do. Governance was properly concerned with employee morale, 9,000 doctors on our various medical staffs, money, tough strategic decisions (identified but not yet executed), external trends and threats in the health care industry, cultural assimilation, and a myriad assortment of other issues.

Amidst all of these important issues, we insisted on taking time out to address a future that was still many years away. From the Board Chair's perspective, she was right to ask those questions. There was enough to say grace over and she rightly needed to be satisfied we were doing the good and proper thing. By day one of our retreat, we had identified the process we would use to explore the future. One of our key criteria would be that we would not even consider our organizational or institutional issues in our Futures Task Force deliberations or research. As responsible leaders, we had to take off the blinders and focus on the critical demands for a robust future, rather than today's burning issues. The Chair of the Board got it!! She understood the need for situational awareness and became the leader and advocate for this effort.

## The Third Criteria for Addressing the Future: Open Mindedness

In our current work at Royer Maddox Herron Advisors, we stay abreast of change and innovation. We are engaged with folks who are on the ground, serving people every day. We hear anguish, anxiety and confusion, the same feelings expressed by our former Board Chair. It was a time of ambivalence then, and it is now. There is a desire to change and, at the same time, retreat. We have had CEOs and Board Chairs say to us, "Just help me improve the bottom line…that is all we need. If we can just fix the finances everything will be ok."

These are gut-wrenching times. Disorientation is the new normal. The unspoken message from the CEO is that if he/she can stave off financial Armageddon for a few years maybe they will be able to retire. The unspoken message from the Board Chair is, "Why in the world did I accept this role," and "How fast can I hand it off to someone else?" Since we are often called in by organizations that are facing the most serious difficulty, it is likely we are hearing messages from those with the highest anxiety. We hope your organization is not one of these. It is our premise that a properly valued and constructed orientation to the future will help you minimize anxiety, get you prepared for changes which in many cases are inevitable, and which will help you sustain your organization so that it can contribute to its community for many years to come.

Having a future orientation requires patience. It does not come quickly, and it does not come easily. Just as a historian must dig through mountains of information and sift it with reasoned judgment and verifiable facts to reach a conclusion, an attempt to understand the implications of the future uses similar techniques. An approach to the future must secure our ability to talk about it without denial. True enough, there may be fear and trepidation, but we cannot ignore the facts that undergird an unfolding future. There are oftentimes leaders who avoid change.

Denial is a powerful force of human nature…. and it is a uniquely human condition. We resist that which is a threat to us or difficult for us, or which go against our preconceived notions of the way things should be. As long as implications are far enough out, we think we can adapt when the requirement to do so becomes part of our current reality. Ideological certainty has no place in an effort to develop an awareness of the implications of the future. Open mindedness is an absolute requirement.

**The Fourth Criteria for Addressing the Future: Trust**

Normally, a time of organizational upheaval and turmoil is not one in which an organization looks to the future. Yet, we were able to develop a Futures Task Force, not once – but twice – and to fund them with time, money and commitment. We were able to do this because of trust.

Leaders are responsible for the welfare of their organization. Developing a better, more fulsome and healthy organization than that which was present when the leader arrived is the ultimate role and responsibility. Leaders cannot get this accomplished alone. Peter Drucker says it well, "The ultimate task of leadership is to create human energies and human vision." (58) The measure of a leader is to create an environment in which others in the organization can flourish; where they can think creatively, where they can imagine, where they can say, "what if?" We were fortunate to have a leader who lived this out, who knew that the responsibility for the formation and ultimately for the emergence of our organization and its success was a shared and team endeavor.

Trust is the product of confidence and familiarity. Confidence comes from observed and demonstrated skill, honesty and frankness with a healthy dose of receptivity and mutual respect. Familiarity comes from shared experiences and a mutual foundation supported by a common philosophy. In a time of uncertainty leaders may be tempted to exert greater control, establish strict rules for internal behavior as well as external engagement, and demand detailed reporting back up the chain. This is dangerous because all it does is preserve the status quo at a time when change, adaptation and evolution are required. In times like these, leaders must be comfortable with decentralizing and empowering their teams. Leaders must trust the staff and vice versa.

**The Fifth Criteria for Addressing the Future is: Overcoming Fear**

Many people, indeed, many leaders get anxious in an unknown, undefined, and uncertain environment. Many mothers give their children a night light in their bedroom to reduce a fear of the dark. Fear and dread are natural to humans. These emotions are programmed into the deep recesses of our brains and helped us survive when we needed to actually run from danger. Without a healthy dose of dread, we became dinner for a larger and faster predator. Something in our early development formed a response and that response has become programmed and wired into our brain in such a way that we will always relate to a similar set of circumstances in the way that we first reacted to such.

Our good friend Dr. Steve Ober, in his 2014 book "Unleashing the Power of Your Story," (59) maintains that our actions are rooted in two things. First, the interactions between ourselves and all other forces in our complex world create reality and, second, we can create our own reality by telling ourselves stories about these interactions. His point: change how we think, and we can change our world-view and therefore, our reality.

Chris Argyris, the well-known Harvard Business School professor, gave us a framework to understand this. He called it the Ladder of Inference. (60) Ober uses this frame to describe how our mind shapes our reality by screening out information so that only data we deem important remains. Not only do we screen and filter and process data so that our world view remains as our mind wishes it to be; we also interpret this filtered information and based on such interpretation we make decisions and take actions. This is critically important to anyone or any group attempting to deal with thinking about the future.

We need information, and we especially need unvarnished information, to build open-minded awareness of possibilities. We need to objectively process data and the blitz of information coming to us in a constant barrage so as to deal with our instinctual, as well as learned, fear and not to be overcome by it. Speed of change has created a breathless quality to our everyday lives. While we may wish to stop and catch our breath, we cannot go back. Retreat is not what living into the future is all about. Leaders have a responsibility to lead others, confidently and fearlessly.

**The Sixth Criteria for Addressing the Future: Teamwork**

In the old movie, "Tora, Tora, Tora" that takes both the U.S. as well as the Japanese perspective of the attack on Pearl Harbor, a scene depicts the high anxiety on board a Japanese aircraft carrier. The Japanese Navy strategist is alone in his cabin, digesting data, sitting under a blanket, sweat beading on his face. He alone is the master of this undertaking. The senior officers, and most certainly the sailors, consider him in awe. His strategic brilliance, they believe, will enable their success. This image is one in our minds about the way strategists go about their business; in isolation, with quirky idiosyncrasies, leading to a powerful and unassailable direction that we must all take to ensure success. While this may have been true for this one military attack, which was considered a huge success, it is far from reality.

In the complex world in which we now live, many minds are better than one; listening is better than telling; humility is better than arrogance. Leadership in organizations must mobilize others to begin the process and sustain the effort. The leadership team, to include governance, collectively must agree on the constructs that could possibly make up a future environment. There are simply too many variables to consider, too many preconceived biases needing pushback, too many limitations in any one person. Conceiving of the future is hard work. It is best done together.

Leaders do not delegate the task of advanced thinking about the future. They participate fully. They engage with a team of people. They learn. They think anew about the world about them. They consider implications. They act. With the criteria for considering the future in place, leaders should use some tested techniques to examine future considerations. These techniques are tools. They make the job easier. They help to break the very broad, sometimes scary, imagination of what a future may be into digestible and absorbable parts of the whole. In short, these tools become new eyes for us to see more clearly.

The Uncertainty Principle and a concept called the Observer Effect have a profound and important impact on any consideration of the future. (61) These constructs assert that the very process of examining, observing, measuring, and assessing, influence what is, and, most assuredly, also influence what is about to be. We have previously stated that the future cannot be predicted. The very act of considering the future alters the future. It is a paradox. Therefore, the only thing that we can rationally do is to prepare for an unknown, albeit suspected, future or futures. We do so by employing time tested tools and techniques to help us.

## Tools to Envision the Future

There are several tools that we employ to help us envision the future and be effective drivers of change.

## Trends and Patterns

John Naisbitt in his seminal book, Megatrends, (62) said that the most reliable way to prepare for the future is by knowing the present. He studied society by using a technique developed in WWII called content analysis. One of these practices was to look at newspaper headlines, particularly in local newspapers. When he found a topic beginning to repeat itself over time he made note of a developing trend based on similar patterns. His journals and extensive notes enabled him to clearly identify trends that were happening all around us, but which few of us could articulate. Naming them became part of the dialogue about a possible future for America.

Clearly, data points assembled together over time can reveal a clear picture if we view the data with a limited amount of bias and social filtering. Naisbitt limited bias by recording only events and/or behaviors. This means we have to collect data, or acquire it, from trusted sources-preferably observation, analyze it objectively, draw implications and responsibly act as appropriate.

Simple to say, hard to do. Understanding the data is helped by extension, the projection of the data, into a future time period.

Let's use the Office of the Inspector General of the United States (OIG) as an example of a data point which, when extended, may be a powerful indication of what is about to come. The OIG has oversight of about 25 percent of the Federal Budget. It has power, and it uses it. It is charged with examining misappropriation of funds and/or the improper payment of federal dollars. It is worth noting that there is estimated to be $400 billion in improper payments to healthcare providers, a big portion of which is not fraud but simply administrative error. The agency has an enviable record of collecting past overpayments at a ratio of 8:1; it collects eight dollars for every dollar it expends to collect it. In 2010 there were substantial funds identified to increase the OIG's budget, and thus its ability to collect the estimated multiple billions of dollars that have been inappropriately spent by Medicare and other Federal agencies. This is a little known provision in the law. It does not take much to figure out that there likely will be significant repayments made by a large number of health care providers in this country. If the collection to expense ratio stays the same it is not even hard to figure out the amount of dollars that will be collected. The pattern projection here is clear: be prepared for increased scrutiny of payments made and expect to write a check back to Uncle Sam. The implication here is also clear: fix the systems that cause errors in billing and receipt of improper payment or suffer the consequences.

**Future Facts**

Similar to trend analysis, but more easily accepted, at Royer Maddox Herron Advisors, we use future facts to establish baselines for assumptions.

What is a future fact? Previously we alluded to historians studying the past to discover and report on the events that occurred. We know that historians, even though they may be looking at the same data and information, oft times reach different conclusions. So, how then can we say there are facts that will reveal themselves more clearly in a future that has not yet occurred? While nothing in life is certain, and there are no straight lines in nature, to include trends, there are some things that can be forecasted fairly well.

Demographics is the best example to use in regard to establishing a future fact about population. We know there are very predictable trends in aging, in births, in disease and in immigration. These trends can be reliably projected to ascertain population size and characteristics in generalized geographic areas. Of course these projections are subject to some variability caused by social upheaval or economic stress that, in turn, may cause a sudden shift in a defined area. These projections are highly reliable, and it is good to consider a population projection as a future fact.

There are other future facts that are more general in nature because a numerical value is not assigned. Examples of future facts in health care are: "payment decreases;" "new competitors appear from other-than-health-industry groups;" "competitors are global players;" "healthcare providers collaborate and partner together to meet evolving needs and expectations of customers;" "technology transforms health care services, interventions and delivery models;" "physicians are employed for security and social expectations;" "technical advances and social demand move elder care out of institutions and into the community."

Some may call these assumptions, or forecasts, about the future. They are more than that. We know from our own extensive, rigorous and objective content analysis of data and an assessment of the environmental conditions in which this data exists that these are more than assumptions. An assessment of the patterns that have occurred in the past regarding similar situations can lead to making generally reliable projections -- future facts.

## Scenario Planning

Perhaps the most helpful tool in assessing a potential future is scenario planning. It involves many different inputs. It takes a lot of thinking. It is best done with other people.

Not only is scenario planning helpful, it is an important tool because it makes up for the errors of the simplistic: best case, worst case, most likely case modeling done in traditional long range planning. Those who are most interested in getting a budget completed on time often do traditional planning. Little attention is given to an understanding of major drivers of change because, honestly, many folks would just rather not take the effort to consider something that may be some time off. However, an understanding of these major drivers, sometimes referred to as critical issues, properly applied and tested, are absolutely foundational to an assessment of the future. In our experience with scenario planning, many drivers of change are identified in the process. It is a great tool.

As previously mentioned in this book, we employed a method called Outside-In Thinking. This process allowed us to consider the many social, technological, environmental, economic and political factors that would drive change. Starting at the edge of our environment, where we had the least ability to control anything, we were able to examine major issues and trends in a larger context. We then moved to the transactional level of our world where we had more direct engagement, and we then asked ourselves questions and considered issues related to our competitors, suppliers, customers, and regulatory environment. Last, we considered our own organization, the environment where we had the most control, and we linked new learnings and insights to ourselves.

These insights and implications became the foundation for the drivers, the most critical issues, of our scenarios. It is advisable to narrow these down to two drivers, if possible, based on selection criteria of: the most impact to your business AND the least predictable driver on your business. Using trend analysis to develop future facts will enable the identification of the most important drivers. For example, from one of our Future Task Forces, we identified that the two most impactful and the least predictive drivers as: a) the pace, distribution and absorption of technological change and, b) the extreme dynamics in both the financial and regulatory environment. These critical factors became the basis for the development of the four scenarios or stories, which we created to enable us to explore plausible futures. Each of the stories were different because they were based on different aspects of these two most salient forces, but each of them incorporated issues including access, ethics, payment, regulations, demographics, technology and other important considerations. From these scenarios, more focused assumptions and implications could be drawn about the future health care environment and to the consideration of a menu of options for strategic action that would be important in any scenario. These options led to the ability to develop much more robust strategic plans.

These techniques and tools can assist leaders in the C-suite and directors of the board to process and synthesize the many variables swirling about them in a complex world. While it is important to avoid analysis paralysis, it is also important to exercise judgment and decision-making based on the best information and thinking available. A balanced approach, including the personal and team characteristics necessary to face hard truths about the current reality, dealing objectively with information which may be outside of ones preferred world view and using time-tested techniques which help to hone a plausible view of the future, will result in a stronger, more sustainable future consideration for your organization.

## THREE KEYS TO SUCCESSFUL TRANSFORMATION EFFORTS

### I. The Expert Task Force

Transformational efforts require a significant commitment of time and people. It is not a one-person task. Understanding vast amounts of new information demands many people making many assessments. One of the most important tasks of leadership is to enlightening the mindset, and hearts, of governance, physicians and others. Transformation begins with translating knowledge into awareness and action.

Large interdisciplinary task forces are recommended to elicit knowledge, critical thinking, analytical judgment and institutional credibility. It is critically important to have a group, properly composed and sized, in order to: 1) enable the appropriate assimilation of knowledge, 2) process new knowledge into credible implications, 3) create potential and realistic scenarios and, 4) establish the momentum necessary to move a large and, likely, cumbersome organization toward a new future.

In every human undertaking involving two or more people there are varying perspectives and even politics. Thus, a strong, respectful and frequent communication process is vital to ensuring that newfound awareness is not wasted. The expert task force enables a robust, respectful dialogue and lends exceptional credibility to the process. A strategic conversation should become the underlying mode of dialogue in the organization to develop understanding and eventual buy-in.

Depending on where people are within an organization influences their perspective. Age, area of expertise and tenure can have profound effects on viewpoints. When considering major variables such as slashed services, converted buildings or fluctuating financial resources, a strategic conversation is essential to crystallize all the moving parts. And, it is ethically the right thing to do. Ensure you are listening to many voices.

## II. Vision

The creation of a new vision does not arise over night. At times, it may require years to develop. It is a lengthy process, but worth the effort.

Much has been written on vision statements, forming them, articulating them and enforcing them. Simply put, visions must be realistic, future oriented and convincing. A well-developed and systematically employed strategic conversation around significant assumptions and implications can lead to a well written, clear, concise and challenging vision. A new vision statement must be based on a shared understanding of the implications of a well-reasoned and credible future thinking process. Without the establishment of a guiding north star to which everyone can see, any transformational effort will fail. It will devolve into defensive reactions and dubious, tangential initiatives that will stir up dust rather than progress. Know where you want to go.

## III. Roadblocks

On a transformational journey, there are many things that can cause deviation, delay and eventual failure. A single cranky board member, an irate public response to service change, delays caused by legal issues, union contracts and even incentive practices can cause a set back. But, the most significant roadblock is the mindset of 'we have always done it this way.' It is a part of the human condition to desire stability. The compounding effect of this roadblock, however, is leadership. If this is not dealt with quickly and effectively the problem becomes a management issue and will undermine every change effort.

Change agents must anticipate roadblocks that can arise from even the most collegial of people. An example is one of our CEOs who undermined a change in direction because of a very strong and personal allegiance to subordinate hospital executives. It was clear that the change threatened his degree of regard by his staff. He was more worried about how he was personally perceived than doing the right thing for the benefit of the organization. Pushback is to be expected. Listening respectfully to pushback can help capture personal sensitivities and insights. If, based on new learnings and enlightenment about the realities of the situation, a change or redirection is merited, make it. If it is not, move on and do so quickly and clearly. If you don't, then the roadblock is you.

# Chapter 13

---

# The Only Constant is Change.
# Don't Miss the Boat.

**"I Don't See the Room, But I See Happiness." -- Sylvia Hutcherson**

This book has been about change, particularly readiness for major transformational change. This is not easy to do, but it requires keeping on and maintaining progress. "The fog of war" is a term used to describe armed conflict. It encapsulates the confusing nature of battle. It seems to us that we could easily appropriate this term to the changing U.S. healthcare environment. Indeed, as in war, there seems to be a general sense that the direction we are going is like stumbling along as if we are in a fog. Like a disgruntled GI, not everyone is happy about it. Others are encouraged and emboldened. Whatever the case, we are on the move…to somewhere…in this haze…and the environment is cloudy at best.

In 2016, healthcare accounted for almost 18 percent of the U.S. Gross Domestic Product. (63) Healthcare is a huge multi-layered, convoluted conglomeration, a confusing and costly hodge-podge of services, multiple funding sources, aggravating accessibility, and conflicting controls with little coordinated oversight. No wonder no one knows what is really going on. We are in a fog. But, we can get out of it, and this book has attempted to illustrate a means to do just that. In any fog, every captain knows that while progress may be challenged and direction is less than clear, continued navigation and forward progress is a necessity and eventually the fog will be left behind.

Let's look back at healthcare in the United States. It is instructive to note that the first federal involvement in health care was not about public health, which would have benefited large populations of people. It was for the express purpose of assisting a narrowly defined group of Americans. The Act for the Relief of Sick and Disabled Seamen of 1798 was the first health legislation passed by the U.S. Congress. Our government enabled a particular benefit for a specifically defined population. We have pursued this same pattern over the last 275 years. The result has been to produce islands of excellence for a limited number of specific citizens, but without ever creating a true system of care that would benefit most of the people, most of the time.

As identified in Paul Starr's seminal work, "The Social Transformation of American Medicine," (64) there were, historically, three distinct shapes, or phases, to health care delivery in the U.S.

**First Phase: A Voluntary Approach**

**From the mid 1700's to the mid-1800's**, 'voluntary hospitals' were organized in communities large enough to have supporting resources. Often these had lay boards populated by well-meaning people, many of which funded these voluntary hospitals with their own money. Some of these hospitals were founded by religious orders. Alongside the voluntary hospitals were some public hospitals that were, essentially, an outgrowth of the old almshouse. Most people were cared for at home, until one got really sick. An underlying interest in the formation of these hospitals was to remove and isolate the very sick and infirm (and often infectious) from the general society. In one sense, this was a form of public health, or as we frequently call it today: population health.

**Second Phase: Institutionalized Health Care**

**The mid-1800's to the first years of the 20th century** saw the formation of specialized hospitals. These were focused on particular types of patients, women for example. They were an outgrowth of the discovery by physicians that it was much easier to practice medicine if the patient came to them, rather than having to make house calls. This time period also saw more rapid growth of religiously sponsored hospitals and hospitals developed primarily for certain ethnic groups. It was during this phase that the institutionalization of health care began to take shape. The term health care really referred to doctor care and hospital care for some malady that struck with absolute surprise…an acute event.

## Third Phase: Power of the Provider

The third phase began in **the early 20th century** and is just now beginning to cede to the fourth phase. This third phase saw significant growth in physician influence and power. This was helped along by favorable federal and state regulation regarding drug prescription and their medical society influence and control over the management of hospital medical staffs and clinical services. The creation of large corporations dedicated to hospital services began to emerge. Some of these corporations were doctor-owned; some were created by the religiously founded hospitals that, over time, began to embrace the advantages of size and leverage in the market. Money became a huge influence and was pursued both as a needed tool for funding as well as the lucre of corporate control.

As the power of science to cure began its own rise, and required huge sums to keep it going, government and philanthropic dollars were leveraged. Major medical centers for research and education proliferated, and, with each new discovery or newly developed and more sophisticated technique, medical practice cemented itself as unassailable and an unquestionably important aspect of American society. It was during this period that employer based insurance was used to lure the American worker. Benefit packages grew in size and complexity and the health insurance industry grew along with it. As the federal government grew to become a more dominant part of American life, it addressed vulnerable groups (disease specific, aging, poor, children, and others) with specific health legislation…. just as it did with the very first healthcare legislation for seamen. The most significant of these were Medicare and Medicaid. These programs focused primarily on the aged and on the poor. As a result of major federal funding from these two programs, even more money flowed into the industry.

A distinctive characteristic of these phases is that the power of the provider was established, and far from abating over time, this power grew stronger. The result of unvarnished power and influence is the growing insensitivity of those in power to the larger society they were created to serve. This resulted in a reliance, and, indeed, comfort on what we are calling corporate recipes to take hold of the hearts and minds of otherwise well meaning people in the delivery of health.

## Fourth Phase: Consumer-Focus

Now we are entering the fourth phase. Population health is the new law of the land, and the fog is getting denser. There is an imperative for change, and it came in the form of the Patient Protection and Affordable Care Act (ACA). Certainly, the ACA is causing significant structural change in health care delivery because of the incentives and financial implications of the law. Defined quality measures, tied to performance and pay, are encouraging an overhaul in practice patterns and creating new alignments to ensure compliance.

Regulations are now in place that are designed to improve access and health care coverage, enhance, or at minimum maintain, quality of services and do this while payment for services will decline. It has taken years to put the pieces of this legislation in place. The most significant change will be the reduction in revenue for the healthcare provider; which, of course, is a cost benefit for the healthcare consumer. All of these legislated mandates and new rules and regulations have stimulated a non-legislated change. The rise of influence by the health care consumer, we project, will be the dominant theme of the fourth phase of medicine in America. It is clear any healthcare legislation will be modified, amended, or altered. Such legislation has far reaching implications. It is our hope that, like changes to Medicare and Medicaid and many other separate pieces of health legislation, as the ACA is altered, it will be done so in a way that actually improves lives and reduces overall cost. We are convinced that the power of the healthcare consumer will require that this be so.

**It's Time For Change**

There are many interesting, but not unexpected, factors to consider for what the next phase will bring. Contrary to what some might think, it is not doom and gloom. However, it promises to bring some profound changes. Perhaps it is best described as a rebalancing of the healthcare value equation. Healthcare value is the product of quality + satisfaction / cost. The societal exemption and exclusionary role that the healthcare industry has enjoyed for most of the history of the U.S. will be altered. It will be driven by the age-old driver of change: money.

Fidelity Investments conducted a study to measure the expected lifetime healthcare costs for a 65-year-old. The study showed that while many things get better with age, the cost of health care isn't one of them. Fidelity's Retirement Health Care Cost Estimate reveals that a couple, both aged 65 and retiring in 2015, can expect to spend an estimated $245,000 on health care throughout retirement, up from $220,000 the prior year. That figure has increased 29 percent since 2005, when it was $190,000. Factors boosting the estimate include longer life expectancies and anticipated annual increases for medical and prescription expenses. (65)

A high number of Americans cannot afford this. The Federal Reserve reports that the health care liability for 44 percent of women age 60-65 is greater than their net worth. (66) Scott Burns, not a healthcare professional, but rather a nationally syndicated financial writer focusing on retirement planning, declared, "Healthcare has become an administrated tyranny, a national extortion. It threatens our ability to lead a normal life. People live in fear of any kind of health event, in fear of changes in insurance policies, in fear of cancellation of policies. People live in fear of healthcare itself. It's time for change. Big change." (67) The healthcare profession has become accustomed to politicians, employers or socially reform-minded folks expressing this type of rhetoric, but when it becomes a part of the mainstream financial literature then this represents a major shift and thus, the beginning of a new phase.

The shift toward the Consumer-Focused Phase is underway. The underlying reason for this shift is not just cost; it is also one of value. The national perception is that American healthcare is becoming both more expensive and less responsive. The consumer experience in accessing retail America is resulting in rising expectations for healthcare institutions. Retailers in every facet of our lives are using technology and new patterns of service for catering to personal needs to meet or exceed consumer expectations. Healthcare is way behind. We have spent our professional lives in the industry and, sadly, we have found our very own individual and personal experiences to be woefully inadequate, confusing, expensive, contradictory, inconvenient and maddeningly unsatisfactory. The industry is ripe for revision. It is coming, not from inside the industry, rather from government regulation, employer focus and customer demand.

## Open Door for Change

It has been widely recognized that at least 30 percent of every healthcare dollar is wasted due to burdensome processes, administrative redundancy and error. (68) This becomes attractive for change agents. A response to this is coming from tech industry entrepreneurs. There has already been a dramatic rise in the number of new healthcare service companies and healthcare software companies. New innovations include software applications that allow consumers to manage their own health, comparison shop for price, convenience and help in identifying alternatives for services, capturing needed health information, and improving fitness. WebMD is now attracting more than 180 million visitors every month. Major companies like Google, Wal-Mart, Walgreens and CVS are moving from being peripheral purveyors of healthcare information or suppliers into the direct provision of care. They are bringing modern, sophisticated, technologically sound and well-honed consumer centric models to the healthcare industry. This, in turn, will bring disruption for the traditional provider.

We expect the main drivers of change will be from continued financial pressures coupled with growing consumer demand and corresponding technological innovations. Within these overriding themes the most significant future trends for the industry are:

## Big Data

Big data is a broad term for work with databases so large or complex that many sources of data processing are needed to coordinate the manipulation and translation of such data into useful information. Healthcare, with its gigantic size, influence and pigeonholed information, needs improved data management. Big data includes opportunities to effect evidenced based medicine applications, predictive analytics for disease prevention in at-risk populations or individuals, and improving medical/clinical quality by reducing variability in treatment and patient care. Improved and uniform standardized decision-making will benefit large populations and patient groups. However, the overuse of large data sets may compromise individual patients needing selective, unique or non-standard treatment.

Due to government intervention healthcare providers have a plethora of new operating rules designed to improve the efficiency, accuracy and security of billions of healthcare administrative transactions. There are newly established and stiff penalties to enforce them. In 2014, Health and Human Services (HHS) stipulated that all health plans demonstrate their adherence to the adopted standards and operating rules. Healthcare data that can be collected, studied, analyzed and applied, is technology driven and enabled. The needed technological improvements in interoperability among health providers regarding all forms of information technology will be enabled by applied big data. It will contribute to the digital tools needed by practitioners to enhance clinical care. Such digital tools can also be used to facilitate patient data sharing. There is a need for carefully developed standards.

The growing use and acceptance of Evidence Based Medicine (EBM), an outgrowth of applied big data and new governmental regulatory requirements contributes to 'cook-book medicine,' as some physicians call it. The advantage of EBM is coordinated care, lowered cost of care and early intervention. The risk is that certain patients may get swallowed up by the data tidal wave and miss out on the unique specialized care they need and deserve or even worse, get exposed by a cyber security data breach and suffer not only from lack of access to the care they need, but potentially to an insult to their personal privacy. Cyber security in health care is woefully inadequate. The industry must immediately upgrade its security capability or the few billion dollars in exposure today will soon become hundreds of billions of dollars in additional costs to providers. We have personal as well as professional experience with poor cyber security. Most health systems are dealing with obvious exposures from malware, ransomware, phishing, and internal threats; but in our opinion the biggest threat is from outside third party contractors who have access to organizational data-but which do not have sophisticated security systems in place to protect the health care system which hired them. Big data is here, it is scary and, at the same time, pregnant with possibility.

**Pharmaceuticals**

Many people associate technological advancement with something they can touch and feel, like a computer, an advanced imaging device or an implant that enables human functioning. In our professional careers, some of the greatest technological advancements have come in the development of vastly improved health enhancing, illness reducing pharmaceuticals. The growing aging population promises to use more and more drugs, which improve their lives and also help them avoid an acute care event or surgical intervention. The growth in the size of the population who use most of the healthcare dollars will push overall drug spending to unprecedented heights. The development and use of new specialty drugs will also drive growth in pharmaceutical costs.

According to a Prime Therapeutics study, (69) specialty drugs, which can cost from $30,000 to $1,000,000 per treatment, are critical for the care of certain patients. The costs are trending up as the forecast calls for a 50 percent rise in the cost of specialty drugs for commercially insured patients. While these specialty drugs are used by a small number of patients the high cost of these drugs will contribute to a national dialogue on all drug costs. This debate is not just about financial implications or medical necessity, it will also have generational and ethical overtones and reflect a growing national angst regarding, not just drugs, but the overall cost of all healthcare.

## Care Coordination

Partially fueled by consumer demand and pushed along by the need to reduce overall cost of health services, improvements in care coordination will become front and center for providers. Throughout our careers, we have always said that the waste in healthcare dollars can often be found at the patient hand-off. We knew this because of our experience in the uncoordinated and unaligned systems of the past. When a patient was referred, or handed off to another practitioner, needed information and even clinical procedures were often repeated by subsequent clinicians throughout the course of an individual patient's treatment. Structures and new models for care delivery connected to payment are now being put into place to improve coordination of care. Models that most often are incentivized financially to achieve gains from these efforts include:

- **Accountable Care Organizations** are groups of doctors; hospitals and other health care providers that come together voluntarily to provide coordinated high quality care to the ACO's Medicare patients.
- **Medicare Shared Savings Programs** are made of groups of doctors and other health care providers that voluntarily work together with Medicare to give high quality service to Medicare Fee-For-Service beneficiaries.
- **Bundled Payments** are financial packages designed to encourage improved coordination for a defined episode of care and necessitate that all providers agree to work together by providing services for the designated or negotiated bundled payment for that particular patient care episode.

- **Fixed Payment** schemes (shades of Capitated Payment) are experimenting with different models that are all designed to stem the rise in the cost of healthcare.
- **Clinically Integrated Networks** are developing quickly to bring physicians into leadership of a comprehensive network of care. These networks offer other clinical practitioners and health systems, population health management capabilities and risk contracting capacity to improve the quality and efficiency of care delivered to its patient population. Almost all new models are some form of a clinically integrated network and illustrate the need for physicians and other providers to work together to improve care while reducing cost of services.

Care coordination seeks to improve access and quality while reducing costs. The models mentioned above may change and evolve over time but the overall construct of working together to improve care and reduce costs will still be a consumer expectation. Coordination is good for the patients and, as well, for a larger scale application. Coordination of care will become more commonplace, but not just clinically for individual patients. It will grow systemically among large healthcare systems, medical groups, insurance companies, employers and government agencies. Continued healthcare cost growth and the burgeoning burden of chronic conditions in our population will drive coordination and new technology will enable it. Coordination will become an American buzzword for consumer driven health care because they will demand it.

**Structural Changes**

Current healthcare models are fundamentally sustained by key structural pillars. These include: licensing laws, regulations governing practice and expectations of care, capital availability and professional primacy. These are all subject to change, but they won't change quickly.

Beyond the fundamentals there are structural changes that may come more quickly. Regardless of the expected growth of the older demographic, we expect to see further declines in in-patient populations. This will have a large impact on the financial aspects of healthcare because of the inability of, or struggle by, institutions to pay their long-term debt. Newly accepted settings for patient care and/or treatment facilities will arise putting increasing pressure on traditional providers. Payment for patient services will be reduced, while incentives for sustaining health status will increase. Scrutiny of objective measures of performance and public reporting of results will be required. We will witness movement from hierarchical structures in hospitals, health systems and doctor groups to a more diffused network style of engagement, an influence model as opposed to command and control.

Consumer engagement and technology come together as tech savvy consumers self-diagnose by using the internet. Worldwide, consumers of healthcare use software apps called medical symptom checkers on the internet millions of times a year. (70) This is in addition to the use of the internet for health and wellness services, fitness tips and dietary suggestions. In the U.S., about a third of adults have used such symptom checkers at some point. While there is still a high degree of skepticism among medical professionals regarding the accuracy of these sites, there is no denying that they are a part of the new healthcare model and are here to stay. New structural models are also necessitated by the functional alignments of doctors, hospitals and their related risk assumption for population health. If we continue on this path, capitated services for health care will grow.

So, what does this all mean?

Many may say that the way is unclear, that the fog of change surrounding healthcare is too confusing and disconcerting, that we should turn back to what we did in the past. We know a lot about what is happening, or what should happen, to improve health care in America. We just have to do it. The fog has not lifted; and the direction is still in question. That said, leaders of organizations can't wait on others; they must chart a path and follow it. Knowing, indeed, is not enough, action is necessary and demanded.

**Fini**

In this book, we have touched on many things that support transformation.
The need is evident. It can be done and must be done. The next generations
are depending on the work we do today. The Texas poet, Larry McGinty,
at the end of his poem Others You Love, in a few words and only as poets
can do, summarizes much of what we must be about.

'Keep a good camp.
Leave kindling.
Others
You love
Follow.'(71)

# Bibliography

1. Barker, Joel A., *The Business of Discovering the Future,* Harper Business, 1993.

2. Kohn, L., Corrigan, J., Donaldson, M., (eds), *To Err Is Human: Building a Safer Health System, Institute of Medicine,* National Academies Press, 1999.

3. Leape, L., "Error in Medicine", Journal of the American Medical Association, December 12, 1994; [1994; 272:1851-7].

4. Levinson, D., "Adverse Events in Hospitals: National Incidence Among Medicare Beneficiaries", Office of the Inspector General, Department of Health and Human Services, November, 2010.

5. James, J.T., "A New, Evidence-based, Estimate of Patient Harm Associated With Hospital Care", Journal of Patient Safety, July 2013.

6. Makary, M. and Daniel, M., "Medical Error-The Third Largest Cause of Death in the U.S." British Medical Journal, May 2016 [BMJ 2016; 353: i2139]

7. Squires, D. and Anderson, C., "U.S. Health care from a Global Perspective: Spending, Use of Services, Prices, and Health in 13 Countries", The Commonwealth Fund, October 2015.

8. Gladwell, M., *The Tipping Point*, Little, Brown and Company, 2000.

9. "National Health Care Expenditures 2014", pdf, Centers For Medicare and Medicaid Services, December 2015.

10. Brown, R., Taylor, E., Dale, S., and Reid, R., "Evaluation of the Comprehensive Primary Care Initiative", Mathematica Policy Research, January 2015; and Medicare Advantage Rates and Statistics, Centers for Medicare and Medicaid Services, January 2016.

11. Sahni, Nikhil, Chigurupati, Anuraag, Kocher MD, Bob, Cutler, David M., "How the U.S. Can Reduce Waste in Health Care Spending by $1 Trillion," https://hbr.org/2015/10/how-the-u-s-can-reduce-waste-in-health-care-spending-by-1-trillion, October 13, 2015

12. Wikinson, R. and Marmot, M., (eds), *Social Determinants of Health: The Solid Facts,* World Health Organization, Copenhagen, 1998.

13. "County Health Rankings Model", University of Wisconsin Population Health Institute and Robert Wood Johnson Foundation, 2014.

14. Makary, Marty, *Unaccountable: What Hospitals Won't Tell You*, Bloomsbury Press, 2012.

15. Schwarz, P., *Art of The Long View: Planning for the Future in an Uncertain World,* John Wiley and Sons, 1997.

16. Subcommittee on Primary Health and Aging, "Examining the Need to Improve Patient Safety and Reduce Preventable Deaths", Committee on Health, Education, Labor, and Pensions, U. S. Senate, July 17, 2014.

17. Christianson, C., *The Innovators Dilemma: When New Technologies Cause Great Firms To Fail,* Harvard Business School Press, Boston, 1997.

18. Harris Interactive, "Attitudes and Beliefs About the Use of Over- the-Counter Medicines: A Dose of Reality", National Council on Patient Information and Education, January 2002.

19. Office of the Assistant Secretary for Planning and Evaluation, "The Effect of Health Care Cost Growth on the United States Economy", The United States Department of Health and Human Services, June 2007.

20. Grove, Andrew S., *Only the Paranoid Survive, How to Exploit the Crisis Points that Challenge Every Company and Career,* Bantam Doubleday Dell Publishing Group, Inc., New York, 1996.

21. Schlender, Brent and Tetzeli, Rick, *Becoming Steve Jobs, The Evolution of a Reckless Upstart into a Visionary Leader,* Crown Publishing Group, a division of Penguin Random House LLC, New York, 2015.

22. 'Humana' 2015, in Wikipedia: The Free Encyclopedia, Wikimedia Foundation Inc., viewed September 3, 2015, <https://en.wikipedia.org/wiki/Humana>

23. Paulus, R., "Proven Care, Geisinger's Model for Care Transformation Through Innovative Clinical Initiatives and Value Creation", Health Drug Benefits, April-May 2009.

24. Freiberg, Kevin, Freiberg, Jackie, *NUTS! Southwest Airlines' Crazy Recipe for Business and Personal Success,* Bard Press, Austin, Texas 1996.

25. Deutschland, Alan, "Change or Die," https://www.fastcompany.com/magazine.94/may-2005, May 1, 2005.

26. Neldner, K., "Complementary and Alternative Medicine", Dermatologic Clinics, January 2000.

27. Kramarrow, E., Chen. L.H., Hedegaard, H., Warner, M., "Deaths from Unintentional Injury Among Adults Age 65 and Older in the U.S., 2000-2013", National Center for Health Statistics Data Brief, No. 199, May 2015.

28. Smith, K., Goldberg, M., Rosenthal, S., Carlson, L., Chen, J., Chen, C., Ramachandran, S., "Global Trends in Human Infectious Disease: Rise

in Number of Outbreaks, Fewer Per Capita Cases", Journal of the Royal Society Interface, February 2016.

29. "The History of Cancer", pdf, American Cancer Society, Revised June 2014.

30. Foody, J., Krumholz, H., Chaudhry, S., "Systolic Hypertension in Elderly Persons", Journal of the American Medical Association, August 2004. [JAMA 2004; 292 (20) 1074-1080].

31. Landen, Rachael, "Hospital Admissions Still Declining", Modern Healthcare, December 31, 2014.

32. Landen, Rachael, "Hospital Admissions Still Declining", Modern Healthcare, December 31, 2014.

33. Ellis, J. and Razavi, A., "The Accelerating Growth of Ambulatory Care Facilities", Healthcare Finance, October 2012.

34. Looney, K., Obrien, M., and Sundoch, J., "Urgent Care Centers and Free-Standing Emergency Room: A Necessary Alternative under the ACA", American Health Lawyers Association, 2015.

35. Grigsby, J. and Sanders, J., "Telemedicine: Where Is It and Where Is It Going?", Annals of Internal Medicine, July 1998.

36. Klein, S., "Hospital At Home Programs Improve Outcomes, Lower Costs, But Face Resistance From Providers and Payers", Commonwealth Fund Quality Matters, August-September 2011.

37. Robinson, L. and Segal, J., "Hospice and Palliative Care: Quality at the End of Life", HelpGuide.Org, revised October 2016.

38. Riquelme, J., "Market Trends Project More Growth for Wellness Industry", Wellness Source, October 2011.

39. National Center for Health Statistics, Centers for Disease Control, *Health, United States-2014,* U.S. Department of Health and Human Services, 2014.

40. Vaugh, C., "The Bumpy Road to Change", Health Leaders, April 2009.

41. Stein, A., "Merger and Acquisition Integration Zen: Brand, Product and Culture", SteinVox, June 9, 2013.

42. Peregrin, M., "Health Systems Governance: Board Right Sizing", National Law Review, November 2016; and, Dorger, M., "Size Matters: Right Sizing Your Board", Dorger Consulting, July 2011.

43. Quinn, T., "Healthcare Boards Seek a New Kind of CEO", Financial Times Service, Jan. 2012.

44. "Hospital CEO Turnover Rate Remains Elevated", American College of Healthcare Executives, January 2015.

45. Katz, D., "Advice for Boards in CEO Selection and Succession Planning", Harvard Law School Forum on Corporate Governance and Financial Regulation, June 2012.

46. Hyden, M., "Are Physicians Retiring Early?", Medical Group Management Association -Connection, July 2015.

47. This quote is attributed to several writers such as Fromm and Hemingway, but most references assert that it is a quote from the philosopher Eric Hoffer.

48. See citation numbers 44 and 46 above.

49. Peters, Thomas J. and Waterman Jr., Robert H., *In Search of Excellence, Lessons from America's Best-Run Companies,* Harper & Row, New York, 1982.

50. Collins, Jim, *Good to Great, Why Some Companies Make the Leap…and Others Don't*, HarperCollins Publishers, Inc., New York, 2001.

51. Gerstner Jr., Louis V., *Who Says Elephants Can't Dance, Inside IBM's Historic Turnaround*, HarperCollins Publishers, Inc., New York, 2002.

52. Collins, Jim, *Good to Great, Why Some Companies Make the Leap…and Others Don't*, HarperCollins Publishers, Inc., New York, 2001).

53. Davis, Alex, "Southwest Got 10,000 Applications for 750 Flight Attendant Jobs In Just 2 Hours," "Business Insider," www.businessinsider. com//flight-attendant-applications-flood-southwest-airlines-employment-2013-12, December 26, 2013.

54. "Curriculum & Degree Information-Master of Healthcare Administration (n.d.)," Retrieved December 28, 2016, from http://www. sph.unm.edu/site/docs/him/degrees/mha/Course/DescriptionMHA.pdf.

55. Jacobsen, Sherry, "Ebola Outbreak in Dallas Officially Ends," "The Dallas Morning News," www.dallasnews.com/news/news/2014/11/06/ ebola-outbreak-in-dallas-officially-ends, November 6, 2014.

56. "Multistage Point-Prevalence Survey of Health Care-Associated Infections," *The New England Journal of Medicine*," www.nejm.org/doi/ pdf/10.1056/NEJMoa1306801, March 27, 2014.

57. Bosman, Julie, "After 244 Years Encyclopedia Britannica Stops the Presses", New York Times-Media Decoder, March 13, 2012.

58. Drucker, Peter F., *Managing for the Future, The 1990s and Beyond*, Truman Talley Books/Dutton, Penguin Group, New York, 1992.

59. Ober, S. P., *Unleashing the Power of Your Story*, Smashwords, 2014.

60. The ladder of inference concept is attributed to Chris Argyris and refers to, the often subconscious, process humans go through when moving from acquisition of knowledge and facts to a decision or action.

61. The Uncertainty Principle, put forth by Werner Heisenberg, posits that there is a limit to what we can absolutely know about behavior of an object. It was first used in physics and asserted that it was impossible to calculate both the position and the momentum of an object at the same time. The Observer Effect asserts that the very act of observing influences the object or phenomenon being observed. It is also referred to as the Hawthorn Effect which asserts that subjects alter their behavior when they are aware they are being observed.

62. Naisbitt, John, *Megatrends*, Warner Books, 1982.

63. Centers for Medicare and Medicaid Services, National Healthcare Expenditure Data Sheet 2014.

64. Starr, Paul, *The Social Transformation of American Medicine*, Basic Books, Inc., New York, 1982.

65. "Healthcare Costs for Couples in Retirement Rise to an Estimated $260,000", Fidelity Investment Research, August 2016.

66. Survey of Consumer Finance, U.S. Federal Reserve, 2013.

67. Burns, S., "Why We Need a Healthcare Revolution Now", Dallas Morning News, October 13, 2015.

68. Health Policy Brief, "Reducing Waste in Healthcare", Health Affairs, Robert Wood Johnson Foundation, December 2012.

69. "Looking Back – Moving Forward 2014", Prime Therapeutics, 2014. A research study on specialty drug use.

70. Munassi, R., "Eight Things To Know About On-line Symptom Checker Applications", Beckers Health IT and CIO Review, October 8, 2015.

71. McGinty, L., *The Geography of Here-Poems*, 2blueheelers press, Houston, 2008.

# Acknowledgements

Every book has two stages – the life experiences that provide the inspiration to write it, and the actual writing.

We are blessed with families that include teachers, who taught us that one of the greatest gifts is to share what we know with humility and enthusiasm. We thank them and hope we honor their legacy through this book.

We thank the many professional mentors who have asked much of us, and taught us the art of being unconventional.

Thanks to our colleagues who helped with this book. We are deeply indebted to Mr. John Hornbeak, a wonderfully gifted healthcare leader who is now sharing his knowledge with graduate students in healthcare administration. John provided numerous and detailed suggestions for clarification and improvements to the flow of thoughts in this book. Dr. Mary Stefl, Professor and prior Chair, Department of Health Care Administration at Trinity University, likewise provided in depth and candid reflections regarding style, as well as additional references that enriched the content. Deborah Charnes taught us 'how to say it better' and without saying too much. Pat Keel for providing a reality check. Ruth Reitmeyer gave steady and faithful assistance in editing, research and assembling material.

Finally, and mostly, thank you to our spouses: Jane, Sylvia and Angela, who have lived this book twice, by sharing our circumstances over the past many years and providing wise and long suffering counsel to us during its writing.

# About The Authors

Thomas Royer, MD, is the CEO Emeritus of CHRISTUS Health and the founding CEO and President of CHRISTUS Health based in Irving, Texas. Dr. Royer has also held positions at Henry Ford Health System, Johns Hopkins Health System and Geisinger Health System. Peter Maddox was most recently the Senior Vice President of Business, Strategy and Corporate Development for CHRISTUS Health, he was the Executive Vice President and Chief Operating Officer of Incarnate Word Health System in San Antonio, Texas. Jay Herron was most recently the Chief Financial Officer for CHRISTUS Health. Prior to CHRISTUS Health, he held similar positions at Presbyterian Healthcare Services in Albuquerque, New Mexico and Mercy Health in Cincinnati, Ohio. Tom, Peter and Jay are currently partners in Royer Maddox Herron Advisors, LLC. The authors may be reached at Royermaddoxherronadvisors.com.

Printed in the United States
By Bookmasters